FAT
NO
MORE

Long-Term Success
Following Weight-Loss Surgery

Gail Engebretson
and
Robert Magnan

G Notes LLC

Dedication

To Uncle Hank. I miss you. I hope you somehow know
how much the legacy you left me as a loving, generous,
kind, and humble man and uncle has inspired me.

Acknowledgments

I am thankful for so many people who supported me on my step into
the world of weight-loss surgery and my journey of discovery since
then: Dr. Megeen Parker, who pointed me in the right direction; Dr. Jon
Gould and Dr. Michael Garren, who performed the surgery and have
been constantly available to answer questions and guide me; Dr. Karol
Gutowski, who helped sculpt my new body; and Susan Reinhardt and
the entire University of Wisconsin/Meriter Bariatric Program staff.

I couldn't have done it without all my fellow bariatric friends, especially my two support groups; Cinda LaMar, LCSW; my coach, Jan
Loiselle; and all my friends and family who have encouraged me and
been my cheerleaders, my guides, and my support.

I'm privileged to have four amazing siblings — Dave, Alan, Marcia,
and Mark, who have always supported me through "thick and thin." But
most especially Marcia, who taught me the joy of staying physically
fit, and Alan, who showed me what it is to be truly courageous and to
persevere through tremendous adversity.

Then there is another special group of people who not only supported my
journey, but encouraged me to write my story and share it with all of you.
First of all I'd like to thank Bob Magnan, who willingly stepped in
when I became discouraged and almost literally threw the project into
his lap. He has unrelentingly encouraged me and kicked my butt to
make sure this book got out.

I'd also like to thank Kristen Erickson, who took a chance on a novice writer and, along with her staff at *ANEW Magazine/Brava Magazine*, got my story out to thousands in south-central Wisconsin.

And of course Anne Connor, who has been my writing buddy, editor, and overall great friend.

Thanks to the Stoughton Writers who encouraged me, critiqued me, and believed in me.

Thank you to those brave souls who contributed their stories to my chapter on relationships.

About the Authors

Gail Engebretson has struggled with her weight and the issues surrounding this problem all her life. Since early childhood she suffered from prejudice against obesity. By age 50 she weighed 330 pounds and began having medical problems due to obesity. She took the big step of having gastric bypass surgery on March 21, 2004 and within 18 months she lost 170 pounds.

A bigger challenge has been keeping the weight off — a challenge for all weight-loss surgery patients. She has been succeeding through educating herself on the effects of weight-loss surgery and changing her lifestyle. She has become more confident, outgoing, and active, spending much of her free time enjoying biking, hiking, tennis, kayaking, dancing, kick boxing, and swimming.

Gail has been teaching violin for over 30 years. She has also written articles for local newspapers and magazines. When she was deciding on weight-loss surgery, a regional magazine invited her to write a series of articles on her experiences with weight-loss surgery. Those articles became the heart of this book.

Robert Magnan is an editor and the author of books in higher education, business, and other areas. He specializes as a book doctor and advisor.

Foreword

Dr. Jon Gould, M.D., and Dr. Michael J. Garren, M.D.

The statistics are frightening. More than one in three American adults are obese. Obesity in children and adolescents is becoming increasingly more prevalent. Obesity causes many significant health problems, costs more than $100 billion to treat each and every year, takes lives early, and affects the day-to-day quality of life of the obese in a way that someone who has never been obese can't possibly understand.

Since the mid-1990s, morbidly obese individuals have increasingly opted for bariatric surgery to lose weight, become healthier, and get their lives back. Data shows that bariatric surgery can lead to significant weight loss, which in turn can result in the complete resolution of obesity-related medical conditions such as type 2 diabetes. The vast majority of formerly obese bariatric surgery patients can expect to live longer and happier lives.

But there are many significant challenges along this path for most patients. Some patients struggle to even achieve these goals to any extent. The early challenges are often quite different from those encountered in the years following surgery, after the weight loss has stopped.

As Gail has done such a nice job describing in her book, bariatric surgery is more than just an operation — it is a total life commitment that begins well before the surgery date. As surgeons, we are fond of saying, "Bariatric surgery is just a tool." We provide patients with that tool, teach them how to use it, and support them while they use it, but the surgery is really only a small part of the big picture. To be successful and to stay healthy and happy requires the proper balance of perspective, determination, resilience, and humility. There will be setbacks! Long-term support and follow-up are essential for long-term success.

There is a lot to learn from the experiences of others who have been there before. Gail has provided an insightful, inside look at life as a bariatric surgery patient during the most difficult times, the first few years after surgery.

Perhaps you are morbidly obese and are considering surgery. Maybe you have had surgery or you are close to someone who has had it. Whatever your reason for reading this book, we hope that you will enjoy it and that it helps you realize what it really takes to become ... and remain ... fat no more!

Introduction

Bariatric surgery is considered more and more to be the "magic bullet" to slay that demon of obesity, the way to be ... fat no more.

Unfortunately, it's just not that simple. Life after surgery is full of changes, some wonderful and some unpleasant. It's an adventure, with ups and downs and good times and bad. And surgery is definitely not the complete answer to the question of obesity. Bariatric surgery alters your physical and physiological response to what you eat, but it's up to you to make the life changes essential to support and maintain the successful weight loss you will achieve.

Maybe you chose Roux-en-Y gastric bypass surgery, like me. Maybe you chose laparoscopic adjustable silicone gastric banding surgery (usually known by the trademarked name, LAP-BAND®). Or maybe you chose a relatively new procedure, the gastric sleeve (vertical sleeve gastrectomy). Whichever the surgical procedure, you started on a journey for life, a new life, a better life.

The main caution for the journey that you started with surgery, the main theme of this book, the primary reason for writing it, is that bariatric surgery does not guarantee long-term success at losing weight and then maintaining your target weight. The surgeons did their part; the rest is up to you.

In this book you can accompany me on my journey, through journal entries that record the first two years of my new life and the many things I've learned along the way.

Maybe you're in the first six months after surgery. Maybe you're beyond that and going strong so far. Maybe you've had trouble here and there and even gotten bogged down. Depending on where you are in your new life, with each chapter you may be learning something about what lies ahead of you, or you may be nodding your head and remembering your experiences at that time point after surgery, or you may be getting some guidance, inspiration, and motivation from these pages.

This book is based on what I've learned from my research, from my doctors and their bariatric team, from the informational materials they provided me, and from my personal experiences and the experiences of people I've met who have chosen bariatric surgery. There are many facts about bariatric surgery and the changes in life that result. There are some rules about taking care of the new body that are universal. And then there are opinions and suggestions and warnings that are less widely shared and accepted. Sometimes the information out there may confuse you.

And sometimes there's no right and no wrong, just whatever works for you. And there's no experience quite like your own. Your new body and your new life are what you make of them — you alone.

Whatever your situation and aspirations and expectations and concerns, this book is intended as a guide to help you through the bad times, the challenges, and the temptations, and to help you discover the many joys and opportunities of being ... fat no more.

— Gail Engebretson

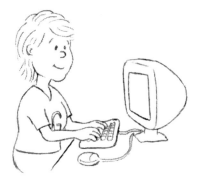

Chapter 1. So You've Made the Big Decision

11/4/03

Today is my 52nd birthday. I've been overweight my whole life and tried so many diets, I've lost track. They've all been successful. I'm a weight-loss champ. The catch is, I always gain it back, with a few extra pounds added on. It's been the frustration of my life, the one area where I've felt like a failure. In the past I wanted to lose weight to be thin and beautiful, attract men, and feel sexy. Now I want to lose weight to feel better, improve my health and stave off major health problems. Truth be told, I wouldn't mind some of the other benefits too.

I currently have no major health issues, except a wicked case of acid reflux and lower back problems. But my family history has me feeling like a time bomb. My grandmother, mother, and aunt all developed diabetes by the time they were 60. My mother died of congestive heart failure, my father had his first heart attack in his 50s and all four of his brothers had triple bypass surgery. However, I did have a grandfather who lived to be 101, so there's some hearty stock there somewhere.

Commentary

We've all heard about health issues connected to being overweight. I heard about them since I was six years old when our family doctor told me I could have heart problems when I got older. He threatened to leave me sitting on his examining table until I lost weight. That made an impression — but not enough for me to do something about it. Of course I was only six.

People who are overweight are more prone to heart disease, hypertension, stroke, diabetes, joint problems, gallstones, and some types of cancer (breast, colon, and endometrial). Any weight loss at all (if you keep it off) can lessen your chances of developing these diseases; if the loss is significant, you can halt or reverse many of these problems. In fact, research has shown that obesity surgery can cure type 2 diabetes.

(Recent research has provided evidence that the most effective treatment for Type 2 diabetes related to obesity may be adjustable band surgery and gastric bypass surgery. In Type 2 diabetes, the body cannot automatically control blood glucose levels. Gastric bypass seems to be the more effective of the two procedures, apparently because it causes metabolic changes that lower blood glucose levels beyond what could be achieved through weight loss alone. But band surgery enabled most of the surgery patients in one study to stop taking their diabetes drugs and achieve normal blood test results. Research on the effects of gastro-intestinal surgery on type 2 diabetes is offering great promise.)

👍*FNM*

11/5/03

After reaching the point where I had run out of diet options, I turned to the possibility of weight-loss surgery. My first step was to do as much research as possible. I searched the Internet for information, read books, talked to people who had the procedure, and talked to my own doctor.

I read up on gastric bypass surgery first — the most commonly used procedure with the best rates for success at losing weight and keeping it off. I also became interested in a new procedure called the LAPBAND® [laparoscopic adjustable gastric banding surgery]. There are no staples and no re-routing of the digestive tract. It sounded good — less invasive and less risky.

The more I read, the more I realized that the LAP-BAND® was not the best solution for me. The gastric bypass is better suited to the problems I face in losing weight — specifically my overwhelming love of chocolate and sweets. Gastric bypass makes it difficult to eat sweets because of something called the dumping effect. Since the part of the intestine the food empties into can't tolerate undigested sugars, patients can experience symptoms of cramping, sweating, nausea, or vomiting. What an ingenious behavior modification program! I need that kind of control.

Commentary

One of the disadvantages of the Roux-en-Y (RNY) is actually an advantage to many people — the dumping syndrome. This is a side effect in which the contents of the stomach empty rapidly into the small intestine. This happens commonly in about 30% of patients. It occurs as a result of eating sugar. The symptoms — profuse sweating, nausea, a rapid heartbeat, dizziness, anxiety, abdominal cramps, diarrhea, and weakness — are uncomfortable, but they are not life-threatening and can act as a deterrent. You can use the possibility of the dumping syndrome to keep away from food with a high sugar content. I have and it works well — especially if you don't keep testing the premise to see if you'll dump or not. Go on the assumption you will and just avoid sugar.

I know I have a food addiction. My addiction is to carbohydrates, sugar in particular. Once I start eating foods high in sugar, I can't stop.

Have you ever gone through an entire bag of candy or cookies in one sitting? I have. There have been times when it's been nearly impossible to stop. You know what I mean. That's an addiction.

What do you do when you have an addiction? Have a little of what you crave every now and then to see if you still have the addiction? That's playing with fire. Like most addicts, I find it much easier to avoid that substance completely. I don't eat sugar. I know it seems like a hard line to take, but I firmly believe that this is one of the decisions I made that have helped me succeed.

If you chose the LAP-BAND® procedure, you do not have a problem with dumping, since your digestive process has not been changed. However, if you're addicted to foods, especially sugars and many carbohydrates, it might be wise to break those addictions. In Chapter 9 I talk about what sugar does to our bodies and why it's best to avoid it.

These are some of the things to focus on before you even have the surgery. Just think of the advantage you have by knowing these facts ahead of time and being prepared. If you've already had the surgery and your focus hasn't been on the long term, change that right now.

How many times have you said to yourself, "If I could just lose a little weight, I could …"? Losing the weight gives us the freedom to easily walk up stairs, sit comfortably in any chair or airline seat, not worry about where we have to park the car, get down on the floor and play with the kids or grandkids, walk into a normal-size clothing store and buy off the rack, and so much more.

We have all spent hours daydreaming about the ways our lives would change for the better if we could drop the weight. How many times have you looked in the mirror and felt sad, unhappy, or even depressed about the image that stared back at you?

So is your focus only on losing the weight? That's why you're having this surgery right? Yes, but if you think about it a bit more you'll realize that you're not doing it just to lose the weight — you're doing it to lose the weight and keep it off. We've all lost hundreds of pounds in the past. I figure I lost at least 400 pounds in my lifetime before bariatric surgery. We're all pros at losing, but we haven't done so well at keeping it off. What's going to make this time different?

You will lose weight following this surgery — a lot of weight! In fact you won't even have to work real hard at losing over the first five to six months, which is known as the honeymoon period. But the honeymoon period doesn't go on forever; you have to be prepared to start working at it after that.

This surgery gives us some tools we never had before. Learn everything you can about these tools and how to use them. Use the professionals your program makes available to you — your surgeon, nutritionist, psychologist, and sports physiologist — and follow their advice. Harvest ideas and inspiration from your support group, Web sites, and books.

Your focus from the moment you decide to have this surgery needs to be on long-term success. Every step you take and change you implement is not just something to do to lose the weight, but rather a step in changing your whole life.

Your goal is not just to lose the weight. That's only one step in a long journey that will last the rest of your life. Put your focus on the long term, on making the changes that will last a lifetime. Take the first step in making this a success to last throughout your life.

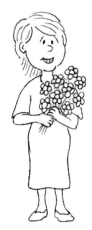

Chapter 2. Preparation, Surgery, and Recovery

1/7/04

I went to the bariatric surgery support group at Meriter Hospital last night. Most of the people there have already had the surgery. They were mostly women, but there were a few men. I was amazed at the results people were getting. 26 pounds in three weeks! 75 pounds in four months! 140 pounds in 11 months! Each and every one was having terrific success and was happy.

Dr. Michael Garren, one of the surgeons, was there to answer questions. How incredible that he does that kind of follow-up with his patients. Some upcoming sessions will have guest speakers to address specific issues. That's good, because I know I'll be going through similar changes and am looking forward to guidance.

The surgery will be performed by Dr. Garren and Dr. Jon Gould who work as a team. I've heard a few horror stories of surgeries done in other places, but never a negative word about Garren and Gould, nothing but praise for their surgical expertise, their follow-up program, and their personable ways. That gives me a large measure of comfort.

Commentary

Most people lose easily and quickly following surgery, but many struggle to maintain their weight loss as time goes by. There are many reasons for this — probably as many reasons as there are people. But there are some basic reasons why people fail to maintain weigh loss. One reason is lack of support.

A support group can help keep you on track, offer you other perspectives to problems you face, answer questions, and motivate you to keep trying. A support group keeps you connected to a network of information, inspiration, and integrity. There is no other group of people who know and understand all that you are experiencing. If it is set up and run well, a support group can provide ongoing information.

The world of weight-loss surgery is ever changing. The surgeons and their programs can keep you up on new information through their support groups. Many programs offer the option of attending a support group, while some make it mandatory for a certain period of time.

It's a good idea to attend at least one support group meeting before your surgery. You'll find out a great deal about the program, get answers to your questions, and meet other people going on the same journey as you.

If your surgeons don't offer a support group or their support group only includes people in a particular stage of weight loss, find a group that will meet your needs. Attend the group meetings regularly. Make it a priority in your life, setting aside that time each month for the new you.

If there's no support group in your area that will meet your needs, start one, even if you begin with only two or three members. Word will get out. There are always others looking for a group that addresses their needs. This is particularly true of people who are two years or more out of surgery. This is where the real work begins and where support usually falls short.

Members can provide inspiration with their stories of success or let you know you're not alone when they share their struggles. They will listen with empathy. Within the group you can share strategies, ideas, recipes, Web sites, books, articles, and much more.

The group can help you uphold your integrity in keeping the commitments you made to yourself. By attending on a regular basis, you are holding yourself accountable. With this group you don't need to hide when you mess up — a habit many of us have from the old days.

Before I had my surgery, I attended several support group meetings run by my surgeons. I had never met anyone who had the surgery before this. I had only heard stories from people who knew someone who knew someone else who had a bad experience with weight-loss surgery.

At the first meeting, I was awed and inspired by the people I met. I found it hard to believe that many of them had ever been overweight at all. They looked normal! Their success gave me hope and belief.

In the months following the surgery, I came to the groups with questions and concerns — and I left with answers and reassurance. I'm lucky that my surgeons are completely committed to their patients and at least one of them attends every support group meeting. This means all questions are answered on two levels — a professional level and a personal-experience level. You can't get more thorough than that.

Our meetings often include speakers who address issues such as nutrition, exercise, psychological hurdles, cosmetic surgery, etc. I have done a lot of reading and research, yet I always learn something more I can use to stay successful.

I try to attend the meetings of two support groups each month.

The first group is through the bariatric program where I had the surgery. This group consists mostly of people looking into the surgery and people in their first year after the surgery. There is always a smattering of "old timers," those of us two or more years out of surgery. This group is crucial for the newer patients, of course, but it's also important for those of us who are further away from the excitement of the initial weight loss. This group offers us two varying opportunities. The first is to remind us of the lifestyle changes that were important to make early on in the program, to help us re-evaluate our commitment to those changes. The second is to give us the opportunity to share our success, the knowledge we've gained through our own journey. This is our chance to give back to the program and people who have supported us along the way. When we give of ourselves in this way, we reinforce our self-worth and commitment to ourselves.

The second support group is made up of people who are close to the stage I'm at in my journey. These people have all succeeded at losing weight, but now are facing issues specific to patients two or more years out. The information and experiences shared in this group are what keeps me going each month and helps keep me on track — some months more than others.

As I reached the two-year mark following my surgery, I felt a need to connect with a smaller, more intimate group of people who were at a similar point in their journey — working to maintain the weight loss.

The close-knit group, run by a psychologist who had the surgery, has become my mainstay, my weight-loss surgery buddies.

We meet regularly and we also stay in touch via e-mail, phone calls, and impromptu get-togethers. These friends have helped me through numerous rough patches and, in turn, I have supported them. I know they're always there when I need ideas or suggestions, a sympathetic ear, or a kick in the pants.

Could I get by without a support group? Possibly, but it would be much more difficult. Do I want to try going solo? No.

👍*FNM*

1/25/04

I decided I wasn't going to give in to the "my last meal" syndrome that always precedes a diet. Those last meals usually turn into a week-long binge of out-of-control eating. I don't want to gain weight before the surgery and make it more difficult. What I did allow myself to do was come up with one thing I really want to eat that I may never have again. A favorite of mine has always been lemon meringue pie. Once, long ago, I had one made from scratch that was sublimely delicious. I've always said I'd make one myself some day. Today was the day. It was as good as I remembered.

Commentary

That last lemon meringue pie was significant and symbolic: I was accepting my new life, for better and for worse.

👍*FNM*

1/28/04

I've gone back and forth concerning telling people about my decision to have surgery. I decided that sharing and support are good. My husband is very supportive, which is great, because I'll have to rely on him a lot. My sister is torn between being excited for me and being scared. I can understand that too. I'd feel the same way if things were turned around. I'm having fun sharing it with certain people, like my friend Anne, who I knew would be really excited for me. It will heighten the experience to take these people along on my journey.

Commentary

My decision to have the surgery was purely personal. I didn't ask for other people's input or advice. I read, did research, and talked with my family physician. After I decided to go ahead with the surgery, I started telling people, my husband first.

My husband was sure of two things — first, that I was going to die on the operating room table and second, that if I survived I would get skinny and leave him. I hoped he was wrong on the first count and somewhat sure he was wrong on the second. I guess he knew me and us better than I did: it turned out he was right on the second one. He wasn't happy about my decision, but he did everything in his power to support me through the surgery.

Everyone having the surgery faces the question, Who should I tell? It's a very personal decision and I think that the answer is often based on who can you count on to support you. You do not want to be surrounded by negative comments and horror stories as you start down this exciting path. You don't need people trying to burst your bubble.

I chose to tell my family and close friends first. My sister and several friends were concerned for my safety. I sat down with them and told them about my research, the advances made in the surgery in recent years, and its relative safety. I then took a deep breath and told them of my deepest desires to be thin and healthy. They had known this as long as they had known me, but I had never opened up to let them see just how unhappy I was and the amount of deep pain this had brought me over the years. My sister hugged me and told me she was behind me 100%. That didn't mean she wasn't scared for me, but she chose to be positive and supportive.

After the loving response I received from those close to me, I proceeded to tell everyone I knew. I even went public with magazine articles about my surgery. I was lucky. In the hundreds of people I shared this with, no one persisted in negative comments or dire warnings. Nobody dared! I think my excitement and positive attitude carried everyone with me.

Yes, it's an intimate personal decision that you can choose to share or not. But it's wonderful to surround yourself with supportive people who are willing to do anything to help you along the way.

We help to create the attitudes around us. Choose to share this with people you know you can trust and count on. We can listen to negative feedback or we can educate and create an air of excitement, support, and love.

2/6/04

I couldn't sleep last night I was so excited. I received approval from my insurance company yesterday and have set a date for my surgery. It will be Tuesday, March 23, 10:00 a.m. at Meriter Hospital [Madison, Wisconsin]. I kept waking up during the night thinking about all the things I need to do before the surgery. I also tried to imagine what I would look like a year, and two years from now. I've never been anywhere near a normal weight, so I have no idea. My mind was spinning with possibilities. My life will change in so many ways. I anticipate having more energy and self-confidence. I look forward to buying clothes in a "regular" store, fitting into airplane seats and restaurant booths, being able to run, not feeling strangers stare at me, and so many more quality of life changes.

I'm not doing this just for the short-term results. I'm doing this to change the rest of my life. My focus is not just on losing the weight, but starting a whole new life as a person who is comfortable with their body and their weight. I plan on making the most of this opportunity to change my life around and put in place habits I can live with the rest of my life. For weeks now my dreams have been filled with symbols of major life changes and a new life. I'm ready, more than ready. It's time.

Commentary

In the months and weeks just before my surgery, my dreams were vivid and symbolic. I often record my dreams; I even belong to a dream interpretation group and the other members help me find what my dreams are telling me.

Several times I dreamed of bridges and paths leading to mysterious and exciting places. In my dreams I was often afraid to follow a certain path or cross a bridge because I knew they held danger, but I knew I needed to follow that path in order to get where I needed to go. My dream group helped me to see and understand that the paths and bridges symbolized my decision to take a new path by having weight-loss surgery. The surgery would be the bridge to a whole new life. The fear in my dream represented my own fears in facing this surgery, some of which I was afraid to look at on a conscious level so they were presented to me on the subconscious level. One of those fears was the possibility of dying, a fear that made itself clear in the following dream.

One night I dreamed that I was walking on a path through the mountains when I was attacked by a band of masked men. One of them hit me on the head with a large rock and I died. But as I looked down on this dead person, I realized it wasn't me who died, even though it looked like me. I wrote this dream down when I woke and worked with what it symbolized. Once again I was on an unfamiliar path through peaks and valleys that symbolized my journey ahead. It brought forth my fear of dying during the surgery. The masked men, well, they had to be the surgical team in their surgical masks. I was "knocked out," which is often the term used for going under anesthesia. In the dream I died, yet when I looked down I realized it wasn't me. I knew that the old Gail — with all her food addictions, fears, and insecurities, hating a body that couldn't move freely —would have to die so the new person could be born.

And finally, the week before the surgery, I dreamed that I was sleeping in the middle of a road. In my dream, I woke to find a black curtain across the road, hiding what was ahead. When I pulled the curtain aside, the most glorious and dazzling world imaginable was revealed to me. This dream is one I will never forget. It showed me there was nothing to fear in taking this next step in my life. That joy and beauty was mine if I stepped through the dark curtain.

Pay attention to your dreams on each step of your journey. Our unconscious can make us more aware of our hopes and fears. We may not be aware of our deeper thoughts in our waking moments, but our dreams can reveal much about what's happening within us.

I saw the possibilities of my new life like the glorious and dazzling world my dream showed me. I knew there was work ahead, but I saw a life I'd always dreamed of. I kept trying to envision how I'd look, but I couldn't quite get there. I had nothing to go on.

But I saw myself running and jumping and moving my body freely and easily. I saw myself happy and comfortable in my body. I thought of myself confidently walking into a room full of people, not worried about being stared at with pity or disgust. I imagined myself buying and wearing beautiful, stylish, normal-sized clothes.

I tried to anticipate how this change in my body would impact every part of my life. And yet, I couldn't completely imagine it yet. I wanted it to happen right away. I didn't want to have to wait for a year or two years. But I told myself to be patient and enjoy each step of the journey. It was a journey I planned to make only once in my life. I knew I could appreciate the results most if I learned from each day along the way.

👍*FNM*

3/25/04: My New Life, day 2

Surgery is over and I'm home again. There was a point in the last few months where I thought maybe I was taking the easy way out of my weight problem by having surgery. That is certainly not true. THIS IS NOT THE EASY WAY OUT.

The day of the surgery is mostly a blur. I do remember the surgeon telling me that I made them work extra hard. They had to make seven incisions instead of four, because my abdominal wall was stubborn. Stubborn? I know there are many parts of me that are stubborn, but I didn't know that was one of them. They got me up to walk that evening. Oh, the pain! But I did it.

By the second day I almost felt normal again. I was up and walking. Amazing what loads of drugs can do for you. I passed the swallow test. I had to swallow several mouthfuls of chalky stuff so the radiologist could watch it go through my new pouch, past the new connection, and into my small intestines without showing any leaks. A leak would be very serious and they'd have to go in and repair it before I could start taking anything by mouth. The technicians were confident they wouldn't find one. They said that Dr. Garren and Dr. Gould were the best. They started me on clear liquids and, as I tolerated them, I moved on to pureed food.

I'm glad this part is over and I look forward to the rewards in the weeks and months and years to come.

👍*FNM*

Wrap-Up

One of the most important things I wanted to know when considering the surgery was how successful could I expect the surgery to be? Could

I expect to lose my excess weight and achieve a "normal" weight? Would the weight loss be long term?

The success rate for taking weight off is high. Most patients lose 70% or more of their excess weight.

The results for long-term maintenance, however, vary greatly. I found out that it was possible to gain the weight back. Though the numbers were small, it was a real possibility. I didn't want to even think of that. I was determined to do everything in my power to make sure this didn't happen.

I decided right then that my goal was not just to take the weight off, but to take it off and keep it off. I looked for books and Web sites that would tell me how to do that. Unfortunately, most of the information out there was focused on the surgery and the weight loss. The information for maintaining was ambiguous and sketchy. I'd just have to find my own way.

The most helpful book I read about weight-loss surgery was *Weight Loss Surgery: Finding the Thin Person Hiding Inside You* by Barbara Thompson. This book was recommended to me by my surgeon. It became my bible. I read it over several times before the surgery and then kept it at my bedside as a reference book following the surgery. There are several other books out there, but I found this one to be the most thorough and helpful.

There are thousands of Web sites that can educate you about the surgery. Most bariatric programs have their own Web sites. I started with the Web site put together by my surgeons and their program. That way I could find not only general information about the surgery, but also specific information about my surgeons, their philosophies, procedures, and advice.

The other Web site I found helpful was *www.obesityhelp.com*. There are several Web sites like this one, but this is my personal favorite. This site offers information of all kinds — explanations of the types of surgery, how to find a surgeon in your area, support groups, upcoming events, determining your Body Mass Index, etc. It has forums and message boards with various emphases, including general weight-loss surgery, RNY, LAP-BAND®, teens, over 50, state by state, plastic surgery, insurance help, exercise and fitness, and much more. You can post your profile and pictures, get questions answered, or make friends. The possibilities on this site are nearly endless.

I used this site extensively just before my surgery and for months after. I still pop in from time to time to see if there's anything new or touch base with members of a group who had their surgery the same month I did.

There are several books I found extremely helpful that are not about weight-loss surgery specifically. The first two can help you create the exercise program you need and maintain it. I read both of these books before my surgery and put the information to use as soon as I was physically able following the surgery.

The first is *Smart Exercise: Burning Fat, Getting Fit* by Covert Bailey. This book provides general information on what types of exercise are best and why. It tells how our bodies burn fat and what we need to do to increase our metabolism.

The second book is *Power of 10: The Once-a-Week Slow-Motion Fitness Revolution* by Adam Zickerman and Bill Schley, I can't emphasize enough how important this book can be. I believe strength training is a must (more about that in Chapter 4) and this is a step-by-step guide to doing that in a new highly effective way that takes less time. And who isn't looking for ways to get the most results from their workout time?

A set of books that address the emotional issues around eating are *Breaking Free from Emotional Eating* and *When Food Is Love: Exploring the Relationship Between Eating and Intimacy* by Geneen Roth. Don't forget — this surgery does not directly address our food issues; it only gives us a tool to cut down on our food consumption. Prepare ahead of time for when your food cravings return.

I tried to prepare myself for the surgery and life after surgery on three levels — intellectual, emotional, and practical. It was important to do the research and reading, but I also needed to start making changes to help support my upcoming needs.

The first thing I did was clean out the cupboards. I threw out or gave away any and all sweets and refined carbohydrates such as crackers, chips, cookies, candy, breads, pastas, etc. — anything I knew wasn't part of the recommended food plan. I didn't want any of these foods around to tempt me. I told my husband that if he felt a need to have any of these foods that he should either eat them outside the house or hide them somewhere in the house. (He went out for meals a lot.)

I then bought a good blender and several protein drink powders to try. I stocked up on foods I could have the first several weeks following the surgery, which on my program was anything I could puree. I made a chicken and vegetable puree ahead of time and froze small portions. I made sure there were friends lined up to help out if my husband wouldn't be available.

I set up a small three-ring binder — a page for each day — where I could record everything I consumed. I would keep track of the amounts of protein and liquids, since it was important to make sure I got specific amounts of these two essentials each day. I also kept track of medications, vitamins, and exercise. In the back of my notebook, I had a grid to show weight loss, a chart to record my body measurements, and a list of protein foods and how many grams of protein each contains per ounce. This became a vital tool for the first nine months.

From time to time when I'm struggling with food I bring this notebook back out and use it again for a week or so. It keeps me aware of what I'm eating, how much I'm eating, if I'm getting my liquids in and what the exercise picture looks like.

Vitamins were on my list of things to prepare ahead. I shopped around and found an adult chewable multivitamin, chewable calcium, liquid B complex, sublingual B12, and chewable C. It was important to have all vitamins and medication liquid, chewable, or very small for the first several months while my new pouch was healing. (See Chapter 11 for more information on vitamins.)

I also tried to look at my needs long term and what I could do now to be ready. I started to put a little money aside each week for the extras I'd need like new (or new used) clothes. Once you start dropping the inches, you can go through sizes every couple weeks sometimes. Go out and get some new or used clothes that fit and make you feel beautiful or handsome. You deserve it!

I would also need a little extra money for workout shoes and I wanted a bicycle later too. I thought about fees for exercise classes I might want to take and checked those out ahead of time.

I set up an exercise program that started with walking to the mailbox and back the day after I got home from the hospital and progressed from there. I knew that if I didn't plan the exercise I might never do it.

The first five to six months following the surgery are known as the honeymoon period for two reasons. One, most people aren't hungry and lose easily, and two, many of us are on a euphoric high. We're losing weight, we're feeling and looking great, we have more energy, and we're getting lots of compliments.

However, there can be several emotional bumps in the road early on.

I encountered the first bump about six weeks along. I missed the food I'd always loved and enjoyed! I wasn't physically hungry at all, but these foods had been my good friends all my life. They were my comfort when I was down and a means of celebration when life was good. Would I ever enjoy these foods again?

We all have our favorite comfort foods. Unfortunately, many of them don't nourish our bodies. You may have them again sometime in the future, but your life doesn't revolve around them anymore.

You're forced to make good, nutritious choices right after the surgery — after all, that's why we make the decision to go through this. It's important to continue to make those healthy choices and start a whole new pattern of eating. Otherwise, why go through this?

Let those foods go. Allow yourself to grieve over them. Grieve for the loss of the relationship you had with food, so you can start a whole new relationship. Don't spend the first six months anticipating the day you can have all the old foods again. Don't squander the opportunity you have to change the way you have used food in your life. Think long-term success.

The second bump in the road was the inevitable plateau. I haven't talked with any post-op yet who hasn't experienced at least a couple of plateaus while losing weight. A common reaction is to think, "Oh no, the surgery isn't working for me, I'm not going to lose anymore."

If you're following your program's instructions, this plateau is only temporary. Bodies lose at different rates and in different patterns. Some drop the weight in chunks, others lose slowly in fits and starts, and some move along at a steady clip for a long time and then suddenly stop for a number of weeks. Keep working your program. Don't give in to despair; it only makes your journey more painful, not any faster and maybe slower.

There will be lots of little bumps along the way. Think ahead about what you might do when they come. I found that getting up and out, moving my body, going for a walk or a bike ride helps. What can you do?

There may also be larger, more daunting emotional bumps further down your road. Prepare for times when things fall apart or a devastating event intrudes on your life and old habits seem too easy to fall back into.

A caring friend asked me one day if I had a plan for the day things fell apart. My first response was "That's not going to happen to me." Thankfully, she pushed me until I acknowledged that possibility and put together a plan.

I built a support network around me that included a few good friends I knew I could call on day or night. I set up a relationship with a therapist who could see me when things got tough. And I made arrangements with a couple family members who would take me in at the drop of a hat for a day or several days so I could get out of my own environment if needed.

I used parts of this plan many times and I'm glad I had it in place. Don't be caught without a plan.

As part of your emotional and psychological preparation for recovery from surgery and transitioning into your new life, it's a good idea to write out statements that will sum up how you're thinking and planning.

Here are some suggestions:

- I will begin to exercise as soon as I'm physically able.
- I will be leaving behind foods that I've enjoyed all my life — but my life will be better without them.
- I will use my body more and enjoy it more for the rest of my life.
- I will focus not only on losing weight but also on gaining opportunities.
- I will reach a point when my weight loss will decrease, but my love of life will be increasing, so I will continue to eat healthy and exercise.
- I intend to be fat no more.

 FNM

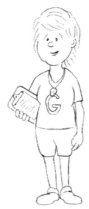

Chapter 3. Power in Protein — and a Few Restrictions

4/1/04: My New Life, day 9

It's been ten days since my surgery and everyone is amazed at my progress. I'm moving around much easier with minimal pain. I even stopped the pain medication already. I went for a walk outside today and the sunshine felt healing. I could feel my body soaking it in. Spring is here. A time of new beginnings.

4/3/04: My New Life, day 11

I was too cocky too soon. Yesterday I felt so good I thought I could do anything. I squatted down on the floor to wipe up a spill and when I stood up I had a sharp pain in my left side. Now I can't stand up without that sharp pain quickly becoming overwhelming. Did I rip something open inside? Did I cause some damage? I was doing so well, now I can't even stand up straight. Good thing I have my two-week follow-up with the surgeon in two days.

Commentary

Expect to feel wonderful — if only because just getting back to normal after surgery can feel so good. Just remember that you won't be as recovered physically as you feel.

Find out from the doctor in advance what pains to expect and what activities and actions to avoid and even how to move. Write these things down — and then post the information where you'll be reminded. It's easy to forget — and you can pay the price in pain and preoccupation.

👍 *FNM*

4/5/04: My New Life, day 13

I had my two-week follow-up today. I told Dr. Gould about the pain, waiting to hear the worst. He said that intense pain on the left side is a common complaint. The left side is where they make the largest incision; it may look small on the outside, but it's at least twice as big on the inside. This is where they insert the large instruments, like the stapler. I may have pulled a stitch and caught a nerve or else scar tissue is growing over a nerve. He said to keep moving and walking and it should work its way out and, if it didn't within a couple weeks, to give him a call. I was relieved to hear it wasn't anything serious. I was also happy to hear that I'd lost 17 pounds so far.

Commentary

Consult with your surgeon, in person or by phone, if you experience anything you don't expect or if you have any questions about what's OK to do and what you should avoid doing. It's best to be cautious and check everything out. Don't hesitate because you feel like you're bothering the doctor.

Surgeons do more than wield scalpels. They should also provide information before the procedure and follow-up care. In some important ways, your surgeon will know your new body better than you do.

FNM

4/7/04: My New Life, day 15

I took my doctor's advice and kept moving, walking through the pain, and it's slowly going away. What a relief! My biggest challenge now is eating. How often have I ever been able to say that in my life? I'm not hungry. I have no interest in food. When I do eat, which is supposed to happen six times a day, I can only manage to get down $1/4$ to $1/3$ of a cup of food. It doesn't feel good to eat. There is a constant feeling of discomfort while eating and after eating. I wonder if that will ever go away.

My current diet consists of protein drinks, sugar-free pudding, sugar-free Popsicles, yogurt, mashed potatoes, fat-free refried beans, hot cereal, pureed soups, applesauce, and an assortment of pureed meat (chicken, turkey, fish). It's amazing how changing the texture of food, i.e., pureeing it, also changes the taste — and usually not for the better.

I'd rather eat soft foods like applesauce and mashed potatoes, but I understand the importance of protein, especially at this stage. I am eating so little and my body needs the protein to heal, rebuild tissue, and keep me strong. So I eat the protein first and, if I do eat the applesauce or mashed potatoes, I add protein powder.

Commentary

It's odd not to feel hungry. You may feel relieved, even joyful that your appetite is not controlling your life. Your new body is different. And one of those differences is that you'll have to think more about maintaining it.

Our bodies need protein to maintain healthy cells and grow muscles. It's perhaps the most important component of our diets. Protein is broken down into 20 basic amino acids. Our bodies combine these amino acids into thousands of protein structures to produce cells of all kinds — skin, muscles, hair, and so on. If we don't get enough protein in our diets, our bodies cannot maintain healthy tissue. One of the common complaints somewhere between the fourth and eighth months following surgery is hair loss. There are several theories as to why this happens, but it seems to be due to a combination of low consumption of protein and the amount of stress our bodies are undergoing.

Protein also provides energy. We can get energy from carbohydrates — but there's a big difference between carbohydrates and protein. Here's how carbohydrates work.

Carbohydrates are sugar, in terms of the chemistry. Carbohydrates such as flour and rice and potatoes may not taste sweet like granulated sugar, brown sugar, corn syrup, and so on, but the basic building block of a carbohydrate is a sugar molecule. So, starches such as flour and rice and potatoes are essentially chains of sugar molecules, some containing hundreds of sugars.

Our digestive system handles all carbohydrates in much the same way. It breaks down carbohydrates into single sugar molecules, so they're small enough to enter into our bloodstream. This sugar, called glucose or blood sugar, provides energy for our cells.

That's how all carbohydrates are similar: our digestive system converts them into glucose. (Except for fiber, which we can't break down into sugar molecules. Fiber just passes through our bodies undigested.)

But carbohydrates differ according to how quickly our digestive system can process them into sugars and how much sugar they contain. We measure how fast and how much our blood sugar rises after we eat a food containing carbohydrates by means of the glycemic index. (There are two lists of foods with the glycemic index for each food at the back of this book.)

Several factors determine the glycemic index of a food. Fortunately, researchers have made it easier for us to eat healthy. They've developed something called the glycemic load. This is a way of calculating the impact of a food on our blood sugar level.

As our digestive system breaks down carbohydrates into glucose and our blood sugar level rises, our pancreas produces insulin, a hormone that signals our body's cells to absorb the blood sugar. Then, as that happens, our blood sugar level declines and, consequently, our pancreas stops producing insulin.

When you eat sugar or any foods high in carbohydrates, the rise in blood sugar and insulin means that your body is getting a lot of energy. You feel great! But then the level comes down suddenly and you feel tired and cranky and your system craves more sugar. If you give your body the carbohydrates it wants, the cycle repeats.

Chronically high carbohydrate consumption leads to chronically high insulin levels. While insulin is elevated, you CANNOT burn fat and you're constantly hungry. Also, insulin stimulates production of an enzyme that causes the liver to produce cholesterol. These chemical reactions are why eating lots of carbohydrates makes staying on your weight-loss or maintenance program almost impossible.

Protein, in contrast with carbohydrates, will not cause insulin levels to rise and fall dramatically. When we consume protein alone or with carbohydrates, insulin is released slowly into our system and our energy level is sustained over a longer period of time. We don't have the constant peaks and valleys of energy and we cut down on the cravings. If we're trying to lose weight, protein should be the larger part of our daily diet.

Weight-loss surgery patients generally lose most or all of their cravings along with their hunger for the first four to six months. However, cravings are a fact of life and eventually come back. Some of those cravings are habit (in our heads), but many of them are physiological, caused by fluctuations of insulin levels.

If we stay away from refined carbohydrates (high glycemic loads), we can reduce the cravings. If you have a meal of protein (such as chicken or fish) along with a small amount of complex carbohydrates, such as green beans or broccoli, you'll feel satisfied longer and you won't be haunted by cravings.

⚘FNM

4/13/04: My New Life, day 21

Three weeks since surgery and I'm down 22 pounds! I've been walking every day. I only walk ten minutes at a time, but I'm getting faster. I have to remember to carry a water bottle with me at all times, especially when walking.

4/20/04: My New Life, day 28

One month ago today was my surgery. I've come a long way. I'm back to teaching and all my regular activities. I have most of my energy back, but occasionally need a quick nap before I start teaching in the afternoon. I've started eating some soft foods that aren't pureed, like fish and cottage cheese and string cheese. I still feel some discomfort when eating and have to be very careful to stop as soon as I start to feel full. If I eat too much, or the food isn't moist enough, it seems to get stuck and sit like a ball at the bottom of my throat. I've found a few foods that don't agree with me anymore — peanut butter, veal, eggs, and carrots so far. The peanut butter caused an evening of intense discomfort.

Commentary

Be sensitive to foods, as if you were eating each one for the first time in your life — because in a way that's what you're doing. Try foods carefully, one at a time, so you can determine if your new stomach is intolerant of any of them. If a food causes discomfort or any other negative reactions, wait before trying it again.

Keep a journal and record any foods that cause negative reactions. Note any differences in reactions; sometimes the way you react to a specific food might be because you ate it with another food or because you were stressed out or because you were too hungry. Foods you've eaten and enjoyed (too much!) for years may act in unfamiliar ways with your new body.

Nap if you feel tired. Your new body will require some adjustments.

👍*FNM*

4/27/04: My New Life, day 35

Five weeks out and down 29 pounds. I'm under 300! My husband constantly comments on the changes he sees — bless his dear soul. A few people have commented on how my face has slimmed down. Most people can't see the overall change yet. They usually can't until I've lost 50 pounds or more. But I can tell the difference. I've already gone down almost two clothing sizes. The more important change is that I have very little pain in my hips when I stand and walk now. I walk faster and with more ease, fit into chairs with arms again, don't constantly calculate how far I'll have to walk to get somewhere, don't puff when walking up stairs, and feel lighter and more flexible. Life is good.

Commentary

Every bariatric program has specific eating guidelines for their patients. These guidelines can sometimes vary greatly so it's important to always ask if you have any questions concerning what you can eat when. You will hear other patients talking about what they are eating and what works for them. You can often pick up good tips and hints of foods, new protein drinks or ways to prepare tasty dishes, but you should be aware that what others can eat and what you can eat may be different either because you're on a different program or you're in a different place on the timetable of what's allowed.

On the RD411.com Web site (*www.rd411.com/article.php?ID=17*) are some very specific dietary guidelines for weight-loss surgery patients from one day after surgery up to six months after surgery. It includes both RNY and LAP-BAND® procedures. These are general guidelines that can be helpful, but they should never replace any specific instructions given by your own surgeon.

It's great when people around you notice that you're shrinking. Comments can really boost your willpower. I knew that from the times I'd lost weight in the past.

But if people don't say anything about the weight you're losing, don't worry. You need to have enough motivation within yourself. That's what matters — you. You'll know you're making progress — by the scale, by your clothes, by your energy, by the lack of pain. Yes, life will be good — and keep getting better.

👍*FNM*

Wrap-Up

It's odd not to feel hungry. You may feel relieved, even joyful that your appetite is not controlling your life. Your new body is different. And one of those differences is that you'll have to think more about maintaining it.

One of the parts of maintenance is getting in the amount of protein your body needs. Protein is especially important to weight-loss surgery patients in the first year following the surgery. Our new stomachs can only hold very small amounts at a time and calorie intake averages anywhere from 500 to 1000 a day. So it's extremely important to consume proteins first in order to get enough of what our body needs.

Following the mantra "protein first" will not only ensure good health and high energy, but also keep you on the path of long-term success. It will be of primary importance to push protein all along your journey, not just during that first year. This is especially true if you find that the amount of food you can eat at one sitting is increasing. Protein fills our stomachs faster and we feel full sooner. Look at what you're consuming in a meal if the amount is increasing. Yes, you need a balanced diet of protein, carbohydrates such as fruits and vegetables, and whole grains, but keep the emphasis on protein. Remember: protein first and foremost and you'll cut back on quantity and cravings.

Proteins are compounds made of amino acids. Each protein has a unique sequence of amino acids. 20 amino acids are considered standard. Nine amino acids are generally regarded as essential for humans. We need a balance of essential amino acids to get the most benefit from the proteins we eat.

It's easiest to maintain this balance if we eat complete proteins (whole proteins) — any proteins that contain all of the essential amino acids. All animal proteins are complete: meat, seafood, eggs, and dairy. Some plants also contain complete proteins, including soy. We can get all the essential amino acids from plant sources, even on strict vegetarian diets, if we balance our foods.

Immediately after bariatric surgery, we need adequate protein to promote proper healing. Then, for the rest of our lives, we want to get enough protein to build and maintain our muscle and lose fat. It makes sense, of course, to choose sources of protein that contain the least fat and fewest calories.

Research has indicated that proteins are more effective than carbohydrates and fats at suppressing ghrelin, a hormone secreted by the stomach that stimulates appetite. Suppression of ghrelin is one of the ways that our appetite lessens as we begin to eat and become sated. Proteins suppress ghrelin best in terms of the combination of depth and duration of suppression. Fats—surprise!—suppress ghrelin quite poorly. Carbohydrates are very effective at suppressing ghrelin at first, but then the levels of ghrelin rebound and rise even higher.

You may need a new attitude toward food, a new approach to eating. Food cannot be the enemy; food can be something you enjoy appropriately. Food will be nutrition: it will be important to know what your body needs and why, because you will have to take better care of it.

Some of the behaviors that you'll need to adopt to lose weight after surgery are different from behaviors you may have tried to lose weight in the past.

- Maybe you've tried for years to eat less often. Now you may need to eat more frequently.

- Maybe you've been trying to drink more water so you will eat less. Now it's better not to drink while you're eating, to wait 30 minutes after you finish eating.

- Maybe you've spent years eating foods low in calories — foods that may have been high in "readily available" carbohydrates, such as rice cakes and popcorn. Now you've got to accept the fact that many of those low-calorie foods have high glycemic indexes and you should avoid eating them.

- Maybe you've eaten more filling foods, including fruits and vegetables, in order to reduce your intake of foods that are richer, denser in calories. Now you will have to be very careful about carbohydrates — including some fruits and vegetables — and avoid foods that fill you up but don't provide the nutrition you need.

- Maybe you've been diligent about consuming at least minimum amounts of dietary fiber recommended by the FDA or other experts. Now you will need to avoid foods that are high in fiber residue, such as orange pulp, and some fruits and vegetables with skin, including apples, pears, and cucumbers, at least for a while, since the fiber could obstruct the opening of your stomach.

- Maybe you've developed a loathing for food, hoping to discourage your taste buds from enjoying what you eat. Now you will be encouraged to enjoy as much as possible what you eat, so you eat less.

- Maybe you've tried spending less time around the table, so you'd eat less. Now you may be taking longer to eat.

You'll need to change other eating behaviors. A big change for some people is that you should avoid using straws. The problem for gastric bypass patients is that a straw can allow them to drink large amounts of fluid without realizing it and fill their stomach pouches to excess. In addition, whether the surgery is RNY or LAP-BAND®, a straw can allow patients to swallow air, which can cause discomfort.

There will also be changes in your diet, of course.

If you've chosen the RNY surgery, avoid or minimize your intake of the following, to prevent dumping syndrome:

- Sugar and foods containing sugars — granulated sugar, brown sugar, honey, powdered sugar, syrup, molasses, candy, jelly, jam, preserves, and most desserts

- Sweetened beverages — including regular soft drinks, drink mixes, fruit punch, and fruit coolers — and even undiluted fruit juice

- Beverages containing caffeine, such as coffee, tea, or chocolate

- Citrus fruit or juices, such as orange, grapefruit, lemon, or lime

- Alcohol

You will have to be diligent about reading the labels of the foods you buy and asking in restaurants about foods you're considering ordering. Many processed foods contain high-fructose corn syrup. Be careful about ingredients ending in -ose, such as glucose, fructose, sucrose, lactose, maltose, and dextrose; these are all sugars.

Caffeine can be a problem, as it can cause dehydration and can stimulate the bowels, causing cramps or diarrhea. Because of the diuretic effect of caffeine, if you drink coffee or tea, drink equal amounts of water.

If you've had LAP-BAND® surgery, you may feel nauseated during the first six weeks if you drink acidic juices, like orange, grapefruit, and lemon.

After any weight-loss surgery, you're likely to be unable or less able to tolerate carbonation. Carbonated drinks can cause gas, bloating, and pain.

If you've had gastric bypass surgery and choose to drink alcohol, be aware that the procedure may make you more sensitive to alcohol by changing the rate at which your body absorbs or metabolizes it. This could significantly increase the risk for alcohol toxicity.

If you've had gastric bypass surgery, you may be unable to digest lactose (milk sugar, found in dairy products). This happens if your body is not making enough lactase, which is the enzyme needed to digest lactose. Lactase is produced by the cells that line the small intestine. The symptoms of lactose intolerance include abdominal cramps, bloating, flatulence, and diarrhea. If you become lactose intolerant, you may have to switch from dairy products to soy products or try enzyme products such as LACTAID®. In many people who undergo gastric surgery, lactose intolerance is only temporary. Also, the bowel also tends to adapt over time, so lactose intolerance is generally less of a problem six months after surgery.

Red meats commonly cause problems, because they're high in muscle fiber. Chew them very carefully.

It may seem like there are a lot of restrictions with your new body. It's true. (There are fewer as time passes.) But consider — again — the many even more serious restrictions of being overweight. I will simply mention that thousands of people like me have adjusted well to life after surgery, to our new bodies.

Members of your support group(s) can offer suggestions for eating better. As I said in Chapter 2, members of my support group share their recipes. There are also books and articles on eating after bariatric surgery. I would recommend the following books:

Before and After: Living and Eating Well After Weight-Loss Surgery by Susan Maria Leach (William Morrow Cookbooks, revised edition, 2004)

Eating Well After Weight Loss Surgery: Over 140 Delicious Low-Fat High-Protein Recipes to Enjoy in the Weeks, Months and Years After Surgery by Patt Levine and Michele Bontempo-Saray (Marlowe & Company, 2004)

Recipes for Life After Weight-Loss Surgery: Delicious Dishes for Nourishing the New You by Margaret Furtado and Lynette Schultz (Fair Winds Press, 2007)

Cookin' for Weight Loss Surgery Patients by Dick Stucki (Bonneville Publishing Co., 2005)

Also, as you'd expect, there are dozens and maybe hundreds of Web sites with information and suggestions about how your new body can enjoy food. I'd recommend the following sites:

ObesityHelp Nutrition Forum *www.obesityhelp.com/ forums/nutrition*

Living Well After WLS *www.livingafterwls.com/ Recipes.html*

So, eat well!

👍*FNM*

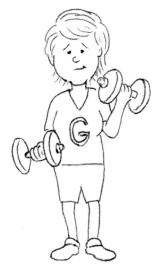

Chapter 4. Build Those Fat-Burning Muscles

5/3/04: My New Life, day 41

Time for my six-week checkup with Dr. Garren. He's pleased with my recovery and has given the OK to add more solid foods and start weight training. I wanted to start the weight training as soon as possible so I can build muscle to help burn fat.

Commentary

This is very important. Put your body to work. Get your muscles to help your willpower lose the weight.

Let's pause for 60 seconds of science.

Muscle tissue burns 70% of the fat that your body uses. So it's simple – gain muscle, lose fat.

Also keep in mind the following scientific fact: muscle weighs more than fat. So, if you're working out and adding muscle, your weight might stay the same or even go up a little at times. Don't worry about the scale. The important thing is you'll see a difference in your body when you look in the mirror. You'll see more definition and tone and your clothes will fit better.

Here's a final fact: when you lose weight through dieting alone, as much as 10% to 20% of those pounds you lose are muscle.

So, let's sum up. You want to build muscle for four reasons:

• to burn fat

• to gain strength and ability to use your body in more ways

• to give your body tone and definition

• to replace the muscle you're losing as you lose weight

Muscles are good for your body. Pound for pound, they do much more for you than that fat you've been carrying around for years.

Always keep in mind that exercise helps us lose weight faster than restricting what we eat. Arline McDonald, Ph.D., nutritional bio-chemist and adjunct assistant professor at Northwestern University, Fienberg School of Medicine, and co-author of *Low-Fat Handbook*, puts it this way: "We all have stored sugars called glycogens in our systems. They're an easy form of energy for us to burn. But it's easy to deplete the stored glycogen through regular exercise. If you don't, your body switches over and begins to process all excess calories directly into fat, which is stored for the future. ... People who exercise regularly don't get fat, because that biological pathway is closed off by regular physical activity. Exercise reinforces lean body mass." (quoted in "The Diet That Conquered the World, by Donovan Webster, *BestLife*, November 2007)

👍*FNM*

5/4/04: My New Life, day 42

I can also switch to pills now instead of chewable or liquid medication and vitamins. These things all make life easier. So far I've avoided one of the complications that can occur at this stage — a stricture. A stric-ture is when the opening from the stomach to the stoma, the connection to the small intestine, becomes too small for food to pass through. This is caused by scar tissue. It's easily fixed by going down the throat with an endoscope and inflating a small balloon to stretch the opening. This is something I don't need to experience. My newly recorded weight is 295, 32 pounds down in six weeks!

5/6/04: My New Life, day 44

My new stomach rejected an egg again today. I knew after three bites that it wasn't going to go. I've tried eggs five times now. Twice they've gone down fine and three times the eggs caused much misery. That's the strange part, when a food goes down fine one time and doesn't go down the next. Adding new foods is always risky. Will my new stomach tolerate it? Several times now a new food didn't want to stay down and I found out that if I make it stay down, I'm miserable for hours, sometimes a whole day. The simplest thing is to throw it up. It brings immediate relief most of the time. Everyone cringes when I say that, but it's not like normal vomiting; it's more like regurgitating. The new stomach does not produce its own gastric juices or bile, so food comes up the same way it went down.

Commentary

Again, be sensitive to your new body. There will be changes in addition to the loss of weight, including the possibility of a stricture — and the probability, even inevitability, of negative reactions to some foods, as mentioned earlier.

Make a positive out of negative reactions. There's no one food that you need to survive. Whatever nutritional value it has you can get from other foods. And if it's a food you've always enjoyed – and one of the reasons why you gained? Great! That loss is a gain for your weight loss.

As mentioned earlier, sometimes negative food reactions are inconsistent. That's why you should keep a journal of any differences in reactions. With some foods, it's easier for your new body to just leave them behind. After all, why suffer from vomiting or diarrhea or gas? Others, especially sources of protein, might be worth a little effort to understand why they are sometimes friend and sometimes foe.

And remember the lesson I learned here: vomiting will be easier and not leave a bad taste in your mouth. Now, what other guide to bariatric surgery will point out that benefit?

👍*FNM*

5/10/04: My New Life, day 48

I've got energy! After my exercise class this morning I felt great. It's still tough keeping up and doing all the movements, but at least I make the effort now. My walking pace is faster. A lot of this newfound energy is most likely due to the fact that I am now down 40 lbs.

5/15/04: My New Life, day 53

I counted my calories again today and I'm still only consuming between 500 and 600 calories most days. I used to easily consume that in one meal! The emphasis is still on protein, but I'm starting to add a few bites of vegetables and fruits when I can.

I start each day with a protein shake — that goes down easiest for me — I never was a breakfast person. Lunch is an ounce of lunchmeat or chicken and perhaps a couple pieces of cheese. Dinner is fish or chicken in some kind of sauce to keep it moist and help it go down easier, and a few bites of vegetable. Snacks consist of string cheese, cottage cheese, yogurt, goat cheese on low-carb crackers, or part of a low-carb protein bar.

I go to the message boards at ObesityHelp.com often and compare my foods and amounts to other women who had surgery in March. My food consumption is about average for this stage, maybe slightly less. I do feel hunger sometimes, but the overwhelming urge to eat doesn't always accompany the hunger. Often I have to remind myself that it's time to eat something. Wow, how different from the way I used to deal with food! But I know I can't ignore the hunger; otherwise I start to get crabby. Just ask my husband.

Commentary

The rule continues to be "protein first" — build those muscles! — and "low or no carbs."

Message boards can help — as long as you don't expect your situation to be like the situation of any other post-op. After all, your new body is not necessarily like any other new body out there.

> ObesityHelp Forums, *www.obesityhelp.com/forums*
>
> Support and Advice for Weight Loss Surgery, *groups.msn.com/ SupportAdviceforWeightLossSurgeryMessageBoard*
>
> Obesity Discussion Forums, *www.obesitydiscussion.com/forums*
>
> ThinnerTimes — Gastric Bypass and Lap-Band® Forum, *www.thinnertimesforum.com*

👍*FNM*

5/18/04: My New Life, day 56

Nothing in my closet fits anymore. What a joy! Everything is too baggy and makes me feel like a frump. I'm down 47 pounds! I keep putting off buying new clothes since I won't be able to wear them very long. I'm saving my money for a big shopping spree when I reach my goal.

What is my goal? Good question. I'm not real sure yet, but I'll know it when I get there. We are told that the average bariatric surgery patient can expect to lose 80% of their excess weight. Many people aren't satisfied with that and work hard at exercising so they can lose 100% of their excess weight. Rarely have I been considered average, so I'm hoping to beat the odds. That still seems completely unreal to me, but I know I can do it!

Commentary

I put off shopping for new clothes. But that's just me, my decision. You may want to celebrate a milestone with a new outfit — especially if you've been dressing "big and baggy and drab" for a long time.

Don't always focus on weight goals. It's smart to set physical goals, such as walking two miles or biking five miles. Focus also on physical ability, energy, stamina, balance, and agility — your new body, your new life.

FNM

5/20/04: My New Life, day 58

I look forward to the days I do my strength training class. I can feel my muscles getting stronger. I did some research on strength training and decided to go with a class that does something called "Power of Ten" or "Slow-Motion Strength Training." The emphasis is on performing the motions slowly and in perfect form so you are sure you're hitting the correct muscle group and stressing it to the point where it will start to generate more mass. The more muscle I can build, the more calories I'll burn. I want to do whatever I can to make my body into an efficient calorie-burning machine — this will help with the long-term success I want to achieve in keeping the weight off once I lose it. I don't want to just focus on the weight loss, but look ahead to what I need to do to keep it off. I'm determined to never gain this weight back!

Commentary

It's essential to enjoy the exercises you do to lose weight — because you'll be doing them in order to maintain your new body, to be ... fat no more.

FNM

Wrap-Up

Muscle is a magic key to weight loss and most of us don't take advantage of that. Muscle has to burn calories to sustain itself. The more muscle, the more fat we burn. Three extra pounds of muscle burns around 10,000 extra calories a month. You would have to run 25 miles a week or do 25 aerobic workouts a month to burn that many extra calories. By adding muscle, you are supercharging your body to burn fat — not just while you're exercising, but all the time!

When you're losing weight, it's even more important to keep building muscle. If you're not getting all the nutrients you need, especially protein, your body will start to burn muscle along with the fat. It's important to at least maintain the muscle you have and then start adding more muscle to help you continue to burn fat for the rest of your life.

Do you realize that, as adults, we are on the slow downward spiral of muscle degeneration? Every year we lose around 1% of our muscle (about a half to one pound) — and I don't need to tell you what we usually replace it with. By the time we're 70, we've lost somewhere around 30% of our muscle mass. Physical activity alone, no matter how vigorous, can't stop the loss of muscle. The good news is that strength training can halt and reverse the loss, no matter your age or gender.

There are many good reasons to begin a weight-training program as soon as possible. It builds muscle, which burns fat; it helps tone your body; and it helps strengthen your bones, which is especially important for woman as they age. According to research, woman who have had gastric bypass surgery are especially susceptible to bone loss and osteoporosis.

Exercise alone can't build and tone all the muscles in the body. Weight training targets specific muscles and a good program will incrementally increase muscle mass without bulking you up. Another wonderful side effect is the way it gives your body tone and definition.

There are several ways to go about starting a strength-training program. Most YMCAs and health clubs offer classes. You can sign up with a friend or make new friends while taking the class. In addition or as an alternative, you can find a personal trainer to work with. This can get expensive over time, so you might want to work with a trainer for several sessions to get help designing a program and learn proper form and then work on your own until you feel you need to update.

Another option is to purchase a video or book that teaches you how to design and carry out your own program at home. You don't need a lot of fancy equipment for a basic strength-training program; a few free weights and exercise bands are enough to get started. I have even known some people to use varying sizes of food cans as weights. We all have cans of food in our pantries, so there is no excuse to put this off.

The most important thing is to start some kind of a program. Whatever program you choose, make sure you work on carrying out each exercise slowly, carefully, and with the best form possible. Poor form can cause injuries or at least waste your time by not being effective.

(I should mention that in the past few years, as I've been enjoying physical activities such as biking, in-line skating, and camping, I've suffered a few injuries. They've forced me to be less active for a while, but they haven't stopped me. I love being able to do things with my body! It's going to suffer a little from time to time if I use it a lot; I'm human, so I have physical limits. But I'm determined to push those limits!)

Earlier I mentioned a popular program often touted by celebrities called "Power of Ten" or "Slow-Motion Strength Training." These programs may seem trendy, since they claim that you can achieve all the strength training you need in 25 minutes once a week. This is the program I use and it works. The idea is to go five seconds up and five seconds down on each movement, which may seem too slow to most people. But the idea of going slow and paying attention to form is valid. The book, *Power of 10: The Once-a-Week Slow-Motion Fitness Revolution* by Adam Zickerman and Bill Schley, teaches all about this method and helps you set up a program you can do by yourself at home.

Women often ask if they're going to bulk up by doing weight lifting. Testosterone is the main factor in men building larger muscles. Since women have such a small amount of testosterone in their bodies, they don't need to be afraid of building large bulky muscles. But also remember, it's those big beautiful muscles that help men lose weight so much easier and faster than us women. Just keep in mind, whatever muscle we can build and add will help us lose weight and keep it off.

Finally, it's easy to feel overwhelmed by all the exercise experts around us with all their different ways to "exercise right." Don't get all caught up in that.

A friend of mine likes to quote a line from an episode of a popular TV show. A character was taking a dance class and the instructor criticized her technique: "You're getting it all wrong." She replied, "Yeah, but at least I'm doing it."

Keep this in mind: whatever exercise you do is better for you than any exercise you do not do.

👍 *FNM*

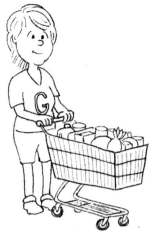

Chapter 5. Food on the Go

5/24/04: My New Life, day 62

My husband and I went up north for a wedding this past weekend. Traveling creates more of a food challenge. I packed a cooler of foods that I knew I could eat, plus lots of water and sugar-free lemonade. I didn't want to be trying new foods when away from home. No, I didn't have any wedding cake.

Commentary

The first six months following surgery are more of a challenge when traveling. It's harder to find foods that are allowed on your eating plan and foods you know you can tolerate. There's nothing worse than going to a special event, letting your guard down, and having something you know is not on the eating plan or something new you haven't tried before and getting sick. Do you want to spend the day of your cousin's wedding in the bathroom? I don't think so.

Early on I would pack things like string cheese, protein bars, small containers of cottage cheese, yogurt, and turkey slices. Some people like beef sticks, hardboiled eggs, and instant protein drinks in a can. All of those items can be easily carried with you in a small cooler.

Airplanes are trickier these days, with the ever-changing regulations; your best bet there is protein bars. Most hotels offer small refrigerators. Check ahead, though, because many provide them only when you request them. If you say you have a medical condition that requires refrigeration of certain foods or medication, many will provide the fridge for free.

When invited to a social event, find out ahead of time what types of food will be available. If there's nothing you can eat, then bring your own. Don't be embarrassed when you carry your own food with you. If people wonder and you must explain, keep it simple: tell them you're on a special medically supervised food plan at the moment. People are very understanding and want to help.

As you get further out from the surgery, it's easier to find food you can eat wherever you go. Most restaurants provide choices of lean protein. Social events usually have a few choices that are okay for you. The trick is not what is available, but what you choose to eat. Even when there are good choices, we often find ourselves easily reverting back to our old ways of interacting with food at a party or family get-together. Prepare yourself ahead of time by deciding to find the protein first, fill up on that, and do not graze.

👍*FNM*

5/26/04: My New Life, day 64

We had dinner at Griglia Tuscany (a local classy Italian restaurant) last night. The waiter set the basket of warm whole grain bread down right in front of me. Ohhh, the smell was heavenly! For the first time I felt a sense of loss at not being able to enjoy so many of the foods I love. I reminded myself that I love losing the weight and being thin and healthy more than I love the food. Someday I'll be able to have a little bit of that bread if I want, but I plan on avoiding refined carbs as much as possible.

The surgeon's office gave me a card I can present at restaurants that explains my surgery and need for smaller portions. (These cards are available from your local bariatric program.) I presented it to the waiter and asked for a scaled-down grilled salmon salad. The manager was very accommodating. I still took half the salad home.

Commentary

Why place yourself in the line of temptation by going to restaurants, especially the first six months? It can be an exercise in frustration. We see our old favorites on the menu and can start thinking about what we're missing and resent the restrictions we have chosen to follow or start justifying why it would be okay to have something we know is not a wise choice. Either way of thinking can start leading us down a path we don't want to take. If we keep our restaurant visits to a minimum, we can perhaps take that very occasional little splurge without slipping back into an old routine.

👍*FNM*

6/1/04: My New Life, day 70

I cleaned out my closet today! I took all my old clothes that are way too big now and prepared to sell them. Anything I make will go into my "new wardrobe" fund. I plan on having a huge blowout shopping trip when I reach the weight I know I can maintain.

I have to admit that there was a small amount of trepidation in taking such an irreversible step. In the past, I've always kept the "big" clothes in case I gained the weight back – which I always did. My head was filled with doubts. Was I really going to never need them again? Others vowed that and yet, against the odds, they gained the weight back even after weight-loss surgery. Would I be one of those who failed?

I hadn't allowed myself to have those kinds of thoughts before; now was not the time to start. I reminded myself that I knew the right things to do to make this a success and, for the first time in my life, I was feeling like my body was working with me, not against me.

Commentary

Sometimes shopping for clothes is just about clothes. It can also be a carrot, a reward you dangle in front of your new body. And your old clothes can provide a sort of comfort zone, reassurance that, if you start slipping back into being fat, at least you'll have clothes waiting for you. If you know that's how you think, it might be wise to clear your closet and dump your drawers. Not totally, perhaps, but at least to get rid of some of the comfortable clothing. If all that remains of your "fat" wardrobe is gray and shabby and made of burlap, you'll feel much more motivated to keep up the good work!

Know the realities — and then resolve to beat the odds. Bet on yourself.

👍*FNM*

6/8/04: My New Life, day 77

Eleven weeks since the surgery and I have now lost 51 pounds! I knew that when I hit the 50-pound mark people would start to notice, and I was right. I get comments all the time now. It helps that I went out and bought a few new clothes, two sizes smaller, to get me through the next couple of months.

Commentary

Even if friends don't notice your weight loss like you expect and hope, even if they are not as supportive as you'd like, even if some of their reactions surprise you and even disappoint you, don't get discouraged. Don't let external opinions negate what you know and feel — that you are fantastic! You look better and feel better and this is only the beginning.

This is a time to be selfish. After all, the bottom line is that you're doing this for yourself, to be better, healthier, and happier. That's the basic reason and you are the only one who can do this.

Oops, I used the word "selfish" here — a taboo word for most of us. I can hear you saying that you're not allowed to be selfish; you have too many other people to think about and take care of. It's alright to think of other people, but not at the expense of your own health and well-being. Look at where that attitude has gotten you. It's time to drop it and put yourself and your needs at the top of the list for a while. You are doing more for the people you love by taking care of yourself than you have ever done before.

Meet with the members of your support group. They can appreciate what you're feeling. Get the support and encouragement you need to start changing some of your old attitudes. These kinds of changes are as important to your long-term success as the changes of your daily eating and exercise routines.

☝FNM

6/11/04: My New Life, day 80

I'm stronger. I have more endurance and more energy. I can do so much more in my fitness and weight training classes. I don't think anything of walking somewhere now. My summer is dedicated to fitness and writing. I've started a water exercise class and I plan on signing up for tennis lessons.

Someone might think I've become obsessed with exercise, but I'm doing two things — making the most of this opportunity to maximize my weight loss and looking for physical activities I can become passionate about and continue for the rest of my life.

Commentary

Read those last few words again — "for the rest of my life." Those words have been like a mantra for me.

Yes, I'm exercising to lose weight now, but I'm going to be more physical for the rest of my life. And I'll enjoy being physical. Why? Because it's not just a way to maintain my weight. It's also because — after years of avoiding physical activities because they were difficult or even impossible — I'm realizing that being physical ... is fun!

I love my new body!

👍 *FNM*

6/14/04: My New Life, day 83

We went out to dinner last night. I've become a cheap date. I either have an appetizer or, if I order an entire meal, eat a small portion and take the rest home for the next three to four dinners.

On our way out of the restaurant, we walked past a woman waiting to be seated. As I passed her, she gave me the once over and then a look of disgust crossed her face. I've had this happen many times before and in the past I usually felt shame. Not this time.

As we walked out the door I was fuming! What does she know about me and what I'm going through? How dare she judge me! I explained to my husband what happened and then said through clenched teeth as my baser self came through, "I want to go back there and slap her upside the head!" Ever the chivalrous gentleman, Bill replied, "I'll hold her for you."

Commentary

A major point in this minor encounter is feeling good about feeling bad.

Let me explain. I did not feel shame; I felt anger. That was a good thing, because I no longer felt fat and ashamed. I was improving my body and I was proud of my efforts and the results I was achieving — even if that stranger thought I was fat. In my mind, I was fat no more.

47

I felt like I deserved to be treated better. As I was losing weight, I was gaining self-esteem.

I would never hit anyone, of course. But my anger made me suddenly realize, in a very visceral way, that I was making great progress, inside and out.

And maybe I should have hugged her, because her look of disgust hit me so hard and made me realize just how far I had come out of years of self-loathing. I no longer disgusted myself. I would no longer accept reactions of disgust from others.

As large people, we have all faced prejudice over and over in our lives. From the time I was a young child and my classmates would chant, "Fatty fatty, two by four, can't fit through the kitchen door," I faced the challenge of being held up for ridicule. Sometimes it's not as blatant as that, but it all hurts just the same. We've all learned to build armor around us — and maybe that armor was more fat.

Society has taught us to be ashamed of being larger than the norm. Weight prejudice is one of the few remaining prejudices that is acceptable. How many times have you heard a comedian who would never consider telling a racial joke or ethnic joke feel quite comfortable telling a fat joke? In the eyes of many people, people who are overweight are weak or stupid or lazy or just plain gluttonous.

When is it finally going to sink in that it's a disease? It's not something we've chosen!

When I was larger I found it difficult to fight back, to defend myself. Now I feel strongly that part of my job is to educate people. When I see or hear people showing their ignorance of obesity, I speak up.

Here's just one example. Recently I was hiking with a group of people and one of the men was complaining about having to sit next to an obese woman on an airplane. When he was done with his tirade, I started mine. He received quite an education that day — and so did everyone else in the group. Several of the women came up to me later and thanked me for sharing my story because they could now better understand a relationship they had with an obese person in their lives.

Wrap-Up

One of the challenges we all face when on a weight-loss program is meals away from home. Wherever we go, there's food. At any social event or virtually any other activity, however passive, there's food. We're surrounded by restaurants. We've become a fast-food nation and many of us have gotten into a habit of stopping for a convenient meal. There are healthy choices now offered at most of these restaurants, but once we're in those places it's hard to resist the habits we've acquired in the past. And when we're with family and friends, it's just as hard to resist eating, especially if we don't want to risk offending.

The other thing to think about eating away from home is that you don't know exactly what has gone into preparing the food. Sometimes sugar is added, which may trigger "dumping," or there's much more oil or fat than you anticipated. (High fat content can also trigger "dumping" for some people.) The safest food is the food you prepare yourself.

Packing lunches and snacks is more time-consuming, but helps keep you on track. Exert as much control as possible over your food environment and think ahead to what you'll need. This way you don't constantly put yourself into tempting situations.

When eating in restaurants, choose healthy but flavorful. If you choose an item that is low-calorie, low-fat, low-carbohydrate, and low-flavor, you're going to feel cheated and resentful and possibly go home and snack the rest of the evening trying to make up for what you missed. It is far better to choose something that emphasizes protein and doesn't include a lot of simple carbohydrates; you know you'll enjoy the small amount you'll eat. Decide ahead how much of it you'll eat (underestimate rather than overestimate), enjoy, and either share the rest with your fellow diners or take it home.

When gathering with family or friends or attending social functions such as weddings, think about the environment. Will your parents or cousins or neighbors be putting out your favorite foods? Are you likely to feel pressure to at least taste every dish? Do you expect to be nervous and therefore eating out of anxiety? Do you expect to have few or no healthy choices? Again, think ahead to what you'll need and then exert as much control as possible over your food environment.

FNM

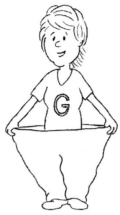

Chapter 6. Don't Let the Scale Rule Your Life

7/1/04: My New Life, day 100

I have not lost one pound this week. I'm stuck at minus 61 pounds. How frustrating! My first plateau. I know all the reasons why this is happening — with rapid weight loss, your body needs time to adjust and keep up, plus I'm building muscle mass, which weighs more than fat. I understand why I haven't lost any weight, but it still bugs me. I put in a lot of hard work this week and I want results — now. It doesn't help that I've broken my own rule about weighing only once a week. I got on the scale this morning, sure the number would change. Scales are evil. Here I am, getting sucked back into the old numbers game. I swear, I am not going to weigh until July 11. I will focus on how good I'm feeling and how my clothes fit, and not on the numbers.

Commentary

This was a tough moment, a difficult reality to face and accept. Yet it was a lesson for the rest of my life — "scales are evil." I will not allow them to make me feel bad about myself.

Do not let the scales dominate your life and control your mood. Above all, do not let them derail your positive attitude. Too much of a good thing is a bad thing. Tracking your weight can motivate you — or it can undermine your motivation.

Remember: the scales measure weight — and that's all. They cannot measure muscle (at least not in a positive way) and they cannot measure how you look and how you feel and what you can do with your new body.

I look at myself in the mirror — in clothes and naked — and I know I look better. I can walk farther with less effort. I have greater stamina in whatever I do. I can lift more weight. And, most important, I feel better in my new body and I feel proud of what I'm accomplishing.

I know what I know and how I feel — and no scale is going to take that away from me!

👍 *FNM*

7/4/04: My New Life, day 103

Independence Day! I'm celebrating freedom of a different sort today — freedom from constant hunger and food cravings, freedom from the ever present worry about my health, freedom to do lots of physical activity and feel great, and freedom from the 61 pounds I have already shed.

Commentary

Sure, there's no real connection between celebrating a nation's war for independence almost 230 years ago and celebrating my individual fight for freedom from fat. But I felt a significance there that reinforced my determination and my pride.

It's important to find significance, to find connections, to find further motivation to celebrate your accomplishments and to persevere in your efforts. So, break out those fireworks!

👍 *FNM*

7/8/04: My New Life, day 107

I am now doing a fitness class, weight training, water exercise, tennis lessons, tennis drills, and walking. My energy level is incredible, which is good because I'm going to have to cut back on my sleep in order to get everything in. How do those exercise fanatics do it? There aren't enough hours in the day to do everything. This is my first priority though. I know I'll have to cut back a little when I start my full teaching schedule in the fall, so I have to make the most of my summer.

Commentary

I may have to cut back on my exercise to keep a balance in my life, but exercise will always be a top priority for me. I'm enjoying my new body and I'm determined to be fat no more!

But it may be wise to get enough sleep. A study has shown that people who slept an average of five hours a night had a higher body mass index than people who slept eight hours. Follow-up studies have shown that sleep-deprived people have higher levels of ghrelin in their blood and lower levels of leptin. Ghrelin is a hormone produced in the stomach; ghrelin sends hunger signals to the brain. Leptin is a hormone produced by fat cells; leptin sends satiation signals to the brain. People with high ghrelin levels and low leptin levels are likely to consume more food.

What matters is not just how long you sleep, but also how well. People who sleep poorly tend to have more difficulty losing weight.

Sleep experts also have established that a lack of sleep tends to lower body temperature. As a result, people who do not get enough sleep are more likely to eat sweets and carbohydrates in order to heat up their metabolism.

7/11/04: My New Life, day 110

I did it — I didn't get on the scale for ten days and managed to take my focus off the numbers again. I lost six more pounds in the last ten days! Down 67 pounds. I looked in the mirror this morning and saw bones and muscles around my neck and shoulders. Wow! I'm not all fat flab anymore — I have a little definition to my body in a few places. Can't remember when I saw that before. I keep putting my hands up to feel my collar bone — it's so strange to feel something hard and bony there.

Commentary

This is a big, big thing — to be able not only to see less fat, less of the old me, but also to see muscles and bones emerging — the new me.

Feel your body. Feel the muscles and bones that are defining your body more and more. This is a tactile form of self-affirmation.

When you're exercising and you feel like you're reached your limit, feel your muscles working to burn the fat, feel the bones they're liberating. Sure, you know the muscles and bones are there, emerging, but actually touch them with your fingers.

I touched my bones and I touched my muscles and I felt prouder, more energized. I felt more aware that I was becoming fat no more.

Wrap-Up

Yes, the scale is an important tool to determine your weight, but most of us know that it can take over our lives. You have to remember that the number on the scale does not always accurately reflect the changes that are going on in your body. Fluid levels change on an hourly and daily basis, an increase in muscle mass can add weight, and bodies need time to adjust to rapid weight loss. All of these factors can change that number up or down by as much as two or three pounds. We all know what happens when that number goes up.

Over and over again the number on the scale can make or break our day. We put so much significance on that number that we sometimes judge our worth as a human being by whether that number went up or down. I sometimes think we'd be better off getting rid of scales completely.

During the period of weight loss, it's much better to try to go for longer periods of time between weighing. If you're following your program and doing what your doctor and nutritionist have recommended, you'll lose the weight as fast as your body is able to. You cannot expect more than that. Trust in the process and know that this is true. Looking at a number on the scale isn't going to make it change any faster. If you're not following the protocol that has been set up for you, then you know that and you know that the number may not go down as fast as it could.

When you weigh yourself, don't let the numbers determine how you feel that day. I know that's easier said than done, but you do have control over how you feel. Our thoughts determine how we feel. It's only a number and shouldn't have the power we give it. Talk yourself through this. Tell yourself how great you look and how hard you've been working. Explain to yourself how the numbers aren't reflecting the reality of the moment. Weighing any more than once a week is only setting yourself up for emotional highs and lows that can throw you off and make your life more miserable and your weight-loss program more challenging.

Once you have lost the amount of weight you want to lose and your body has settled into a comfortable spot that feels right, you may choose to weigh yourself a little more often or not. Then you're using the scale to help you stay on track. The scale can alert you to the fact that you're getting a little sloppy about snacking or exercise or carbo-hydrates. Look at where you've let things slide and decide how you can get back on track. That might be anything from a call to a bariatric friend, a trip to your surgeon's office, an extra support group meeting, a visit with the nutritionist or sports physiologist, or finding a book like this one to motivate you.

Remember, though, if you find that the numbers on the scale send you into a tailspin or a major funk, don't use it. It is better to determine how you're doing with your weight-loss or maintenance program by how you feel, by how your clothes fit, or even by what the tape measure shows. Decide how often you need to weigh yourself — and then stick by that. Keep the number on the scale in perspective and look on it as a tool, not a judgment.

FNM

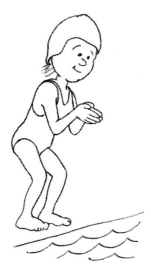

Chapter 7. Fluids — To Drink or Not to Drink: What, When, How, and Why

7/15/2004: My New Life, day 114

Every time I have lunch or dinner with someone, I have to explain again why I don't drink liquids with my meals. This is one of the most important and unbreakable rules for maintaining success after surgery.

Drinking fluids with the meal, or too soon after the meal, washes the food out of the stomach pouch too quickly. This new pouch does not function the same as the old stomach. It does not have the same gastric juices and acids. It doesn't mix up the food, break it down, and digest it. I have to break down the food myself by chewing thoroughly. I want to maintain that feeling of fullness and satiety as long as possible. This signals my brain that I have eaten enough food and I'm not starving myself, so my metabolism doesn't drop into starvation mode.

If I drink with the meal, the food washes right through and I can continue to eat past what the pouch can hold. This defeats the entire purpose of the surgery, because now my portions are not limited in the same way. If I drink less than 30 minutes after eating, I'm hungry again too soon. I'm constantly amazed at how some of the new post-ops on the message boards don't know this crucial piece of information. Either their surgeon does not have a thorough educational program, which is criminal, or the patient didn't listen carefully or do their homework. Educating yourself about all aspects of this surgery and follow-up is so important to success.

Commentary

Part of your new life is learning new rules for your new body, which sometimes means revising or even replacing old rules.

This is an example.

Now you need to keep the food in your mouth longer, so you can chew it more completely. Now you need to keep the food in your stomach and digestive system longer, so you can get more of the nutrients from it and maintain that feeling of satiety longer.

You want to feel full as long as possible, so you don't eat more, of course, but also so your body doesn't feel hungry and react by slowing down your rate of metabolism.

So, there's a new rule: wait 30 minutes (some programs may vary in the amount of time they suggest waiting) before drinking water.

Is this a difficult rule to remember if you've been trying for years to drink more water, especially with meals? Of course! So, when the waiter or waitress brings water to you, try this trick. Put a spoon upside down in the glass. Any time you automatically pick up the glass to drink, that spoon should remind you to wait.

👍FNM

7/18/2004: My New Life, day 117

Another five pounds down! It seems to be melting off me right now. That's a total of 72 pounds.

Commentary

Yes, it actually becomes easier to lose weight — because your muscles are helping burn the fat, because you're acquiring healthy habits, and because you're enjoying your new life more and more and thinking less and less about losing weight. It's so great not to be always obsessing over your weight!

👍FNM

7/21/2004: My New Life, day 120

My hair is falling out! Every time I run my fingers or a comb through my hair, I get a web of strands. This is one of the side effects of the surgery that I knew I wouldn't be able to avoid. Hair loss usually occurs between the fourth and seventh months. I reached the four-month mark yesterday — nothing like keeping to the schedule. Most people experience hair loss after this surgery. A few of the lucky ones manage to avoid it, but no one seems to have figured out why it hits some and not others. I've had hair loss to a lesser degree with other weight-loss programs, so it was inevitable it would happen this time. I hope it doesn't get too drastic, my hair is already fine. At least I know it will grow back eventually.

Commentary

If you start losing hair, focus on three things:

• It's natural to lose hair as you lose weight.

• Your hair loss is only temporary.

• Losing hair is not a health hazard, but being grossly overweight is definitely bad for your physical and psychological health, so a little hair seems a small price to pay.

☞*FNM*

7/24/2004: My New Life, day 123

I still do a lot of walking even though I've found other activities I like more. I keep pushing the distance and I'm getting faster. I have to remember to carry a water bottle with me at all times, especially when walking.

My husband and I went for what we thought would be a short walk in the woods the other day. We took a wrong path — oops! We were out there for two hours. It was hot and I didn't have any water with me — double oops! I began to feel light-headed, very thirsty, and slightly disoriented. I knew I was becoming dehydrated — seriously so. Thank goodness there was a house nearby and we stopped and asked for water.

I learned my lesson. I've learned that staying hydrated is so important, not only during exercise but all the time. Three of the nice side effects are that it helps me not retain fluids, it keeps me regular, and my complexion is clear and smooth.

Commentary

There are two important points here.

One is that I keep pushing the distance. You may not do that. But after years of exerting so much energy to move my big body and feeling so much resistance in my muscles and joints, I usually feel so good walking that I naturally want to walk more. Imagine feeling that good doing something I dreaded doing! So, don't be surprised if you start enjoying pushing your physical limits.

The second point is to always take along more water than you think you'll drink. You may take a wrong turn, as we did, or you may just enjoy your walk so much that you go farther than you planned.

Put a water bottle or two in a fanny pack or get one of those thermal bottle carriers on a strap like I have. It's more convenient to wear it than to carry it. And keep in mind the reasons for drinking water:

- Water is necessary for every body: the more you use your body, the more water you need.
- Water helps you reduce the fluids you're retaining — as illogical as that may seem. That's because when your body is not getting enough water, it naturally works to retain it.
- Water keeps your digestive system more regular. This was true for your old body; it's all the more important for your new body. You don't need Mr. Wizard to explain how water eases food through your system and out.
- Water keeps your complexion clear and smooth.

👍*FNM*

7/27/2004: My New Life, day 126

It's 78 degrees in the house and I'm freezing. When I sit still for any length of time, I'm cold. I always keep a sweatshirt handy. This is a common complaint of post-ops. I'm not looking forward to winter.

Commentary

This is a down side to losing weight, a chill to the glow. However, now that I don't feel an emotional need to keep my body covered from head to toe when I'm outside in warmer weather, wearing more clothes because I'm cold seems like a fair trade-off.

Also, wearing a sweatshirt or a sweater is better than wearing 50 or 100 or 150 pounds of fat, for at least three reasons. One, it's healthier. Two,

I can choose colors and patterns and textures. Three, I can take it off in seconds at any moment.

☝*FNM*

7/27/2004: My New Life, day 126

I can't believe how many inches I've lost! This is even more exciting than the weight loss. I measure once a month. I've lost a total of 27 inches just in the bust, waist, and hips combined. The strangest is my head measurement — down 3/4 of an inch! I've gone from a size 5X to a 2X and am now down a total of 74 pounds. I'm currently at my all-time low for the past 20 years. From now on I am exploring new frontiers!

Commentary

Just as you should not let your scale dominate your new life, you should not become a slave to the tape measure.

Don't think of your body in terms of how many inches you've lost in the past month or the past week, but how much you've improved your shape since you took the big step with bariatric surgery. You're doing more, you're hurting less, you've got more energy, you're feeling better — you're becoming fat no more.

☝*FNM*

Wrap-Up

It's important to stay hydrated. Our body functions much better when it's kept well hydrated. If you're not getting enough fluids, your body will actually hang onto the fluids it has. It will retain fluids. When you keep drinking, it keeps everything moving in your body, including your bowels. Constipation is a common problem with weight-loss surgery patients and it can become serious. A good part of the answer is to keep pushing the fluids. When you're thirsty, it's a sign that you're already dehydrated.

Immediately following surgery is a vulnerable time. Our bodies are healing, our digestive systems are adjusting to the changes, and we just don't feel like eating or drinking — it's uncomfortable. Our bodies can go for a long time with no food or very little food if necessary, but they can't go very long without fluids before our systems start to shut down.

Most of us have gone through life not paying much attention to our fluid intake. We got by because we drank when we were thirsty and our bodies derived some fluids from food. When we're not eating very much, it's even more important to push the fluids. Most programs recommend a minimum of 64 fluid ounces a day and even more on hot days or days we exercise vigorously. Yes, it's extremely difficult to get that amount in the first couple weeks following surgery, but if you keep trying and keep track, adding a little more each day, you can do it.

When you're further out from the surgery, there's a tendency to get lax about getting in the fluids. Our bodies still need proper hydration, plus there's an added benefit to keeping the fluids going all day. When you're drinking, you're not eating! If we sip at our fluids continually throughout the day, between meals, it keeps our stomachs full and cuts down on the snacking. If you're having trouble losing weight because you're snacking throughout the day, take a hard look at your fluid intake.

Dr. Chad Oler, chemical engineer turned naturopath, has a word of advice for everyone. "One thing everyone can do to is to properly hydrate their bodies. We all know we're supposed to drink at least eight glasses of water a day, but we tend to go half the day without drinking and then gulp large quantities at once. Our bodies can only use two to four ounces every half hour, so we end up expelling most of it immediately. We need to sip all day long. Proper hydration could help alleviate 40-60% of our health problems."

Plain old water is your best source for fluids. But, I know that many of us, including me, get tired of just water and want a little flavor to our liquids. There are a lot of flavored waters on the market; just make sure they don't contain any sugar, including high-fructose corn syrup. I like to add a little sugar-free lemonade to my water or drink herbal teas. I also found liquid, flavored stevia (a natural sweetener) in the health food section of my grocery store and I'll often add a few drops of lemon, Valencia orange, root beer, or peppermint to my water. Even though I'm close to four years out from my surgery, I still carry a water bottle with me most of the time.

The other issue for weight-loss surgery patients is when not to drink. Not drinking with meals is one of the Rules of the Pouch. If you don't know the Rules of the Pouch, I've included them at the back of this book. Print these rules out and tape them up somewhere conspicuous in your house.

Drinking while eating can do one of two things. Early on after surgery, it can fill your stomach with fluids when you need space for food and nutrition, especially protein. Then, at any time for the rest of your life, it can wash the foods through your small stomach much too quickly. If this happens, you eat much more or you feel hungry again soon after you eat. The rule of thumb is to stop drinking 15 minutes before eating and don't start again for 30 to 60 minutes after. Then drink fluids to keep your stomach feeling full so you're not tempted to snack.

For patients with adjustable bands, the regimen is less rigid. Paul O'Brien, M.D. — National Medical Director of the American Institute of Gastric Banding in Dallas, Texas and head of the Centre for Obesity Research and Education at Monash University, Melbourne, recognized as one of the top authorities on the LAP-BAND® — presents in his book, *The LAP-BAND Solution — A Partnership for Weight Loss*, the "Golden Rules of Eating and Exercise." These rules are basically common sense. Eat three or fewer small meals a day. Eat slowly. Stop eating when you no longer feel hungry. Don't eat if you don't feel like eating. Don't eat anything at all between meals. Eat nutritious foods. Avoid liquids that contain calories.

That's it for eating and drinking — only one rule for liquids for patients with adjustable bands. The rules also recommend exercising at least 30 minutes every day and being active throughout the day. That's good advice for all of us, whatever our shapes.

Following the rules about fluids will help ensure you'll be fat no more.

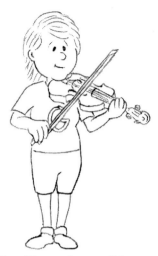

Chapter 8. Raging Hormones

8/1/04: My New Life, day 131

Whoa, these last few days have been tough. I went into a major funk for no apparent reason, except maybe that I'm tired of all this rain. I'm a positive, upbeat person and don't usually get blue for no reason. When I am down, I can usually pull myself out of it within a couple hours, or at the most a couple days. That didn't work this time. It was not a good feeling. I'd heard of other post-ops going into depression and thought I'd just skip that. I read that when there's rapid weight loss, the fat cells, which store hormones, release them, and there can be hormonal imbalances. I was definitely unbalanced this week!

The really tough part about going through an emotional low is that I don't have my old buddy, food, to help get me through it. I've always used food, especially chocolate, as a salve for the soul. I don't have that option anymore and I had to work through the emotions without my crutch. Anyone battling an addiction knows what that's like. I'm sure it's a healthy process for me, but it's still no fun.

This episode reminds me of the times I was premenstrual — another time of hormonal imbalance. It was always the hardest time to not go to food. I'm glad it's over for now.

Commentary

Our bodies are micro ecosystems. That's a scientific way of expressing what we all know naturally — there's a lot happening inside us and all those activities are interconnected.

Ah, hormones! Can't live with them, can't live without them — although at times I've definitely wanted to try living without them.

But as bad as I've felt going through times of raging hormones and dismal depression — I still suffer occasionally three plus years after my surgery — I try to remain positive, for two reasons.

The little reason is that mood swings may be at least partly evidence of my progress, to the extent that they result from my getting rid of fat. The big reason is that these tough times would have pushed the old me into feeding frenzies, chocolate binges and all — but the new me is gaining strength, breaking out of that cycle. I know that I'm not free from depression and hormonal shifts and I'm certainly not free from my eating addiction. But every rough time that I survive without reverting to the coping mechanism of the old me is a reason to celebrate.

FNM

8/3/04: My New Life, day 133

I have lost a total of 77 lbs. as of today. That number seemed so huge and remarkable when I calculated it this morning, but now it doesn't seem very impressive when I think of how far I still have to go. What's that famous saying? "One day at a time." It seems appropriate to focus on that right now.

Commentary

There are moments when you will feel on top of the world. There are also moments when you'll feel like you're pushing the world uphill — like Sisyphus, that character from Greek legends who was punished in the afterworld with the task of rolling a big boulder up a hill for eternity, never to actually achieve the summit.

Unlike Sisyphus, things will be getting better for you; your body will be getting into shape and your life will be improving. But there will be times when it seems like the boulder is getting heavier or the hill is getting steeper and you may need to concentrate on living one day at a time – or just making it through the next hour.

That's normal. That's OK. Just don't give up!

FNM

8/7/04: My New Life, day 137

My body image is changing. The other day, a friend told me that not only am I looking great, but that I seem more "put together." I knew what she meant right away.

I spend a little more time on my hair, wear makeup more often, even had a pedicure for the first time in my life. Did I feel that I didn't deserve that kind of care and attention before? Or is it that now when I put a little more effort in, the rewards are so much greater? I never liked how I looked. No matter how hard I tried, I still felt fat and ugly. When I look in the mirror now, I don't feel total disgust anymore. Of course, part of my self-image has to do with how I feel emotionally. Today I feel successful and productive.

Commentary

Again, each of us is a micro ecosystem. As I lost weight, I took more pride in my appearance and I felt more deserving. It was such an important step to go from feeling fat and ugly and disgusted with myself to being proud of my body, to actually enjoy looking in the mirror and seeing bones and muscles emerging from a body that had been a shameful blob for so many years.

Yes, there are down times, but more and more often you're going to feel the pride, excitement, and joy of creating the new you. Grab those feelings of joy and success and hang onto them. Acknowledging your success sets you up for more success.

👍*FNM*

8/14/04: My New Life, day 144

I leave for a Connecticut vacation in five days — can't wait. I'll be spending 12 days in a rustic mountain cabin with my second family, the Boones. In the past, vacation has always meant a time to relax and be lazy, giving myself permission to eat whatever I wanted — pigging out. Thus, I always gained weight on vacation. This year is going to be different.

I need to carefully plan food for spending a day flying and waiting in airports on each end of the trip. I'm also thinking ahead to provisions for the cabin, which is a 30-minute drive from civilization. I want to have plenty of protein available so there's no excuse to stray from my eating plan. I'll carry several dozen low-carb protein bars, some string cheese, a can of almonds and low-carb crackers. The rest I can get during our shopping trip on the way to the cabin. I'll also carry a bottle of water with me at all times.

Commentary

I felt confident about the challenges of being on vacation, even enthusiastic about putting the new me to the test. It felt great to face a vacation without fear. It was how normal people feel.

👍*FNM*

8/20/04: My New Life, day 150

I'm on vacation! Yesterday's travel day went smoothly and the protein bars and string cheese were the perfect things to see me through the day. The cabin is located in the NW corner of Connecticut, tucked into the thickly wooded Appalachian Mountains. No electricity, no phone — back to nature.

The Boones had invited me to their cabin before, but I turned them down since cabin life involved lots of walking, hiking, swimming, and various other physical activities. I'd previously shied away from those things, knowing I couldn't keep up. This time I'm excited about doing it all! I weighed myself yesterday before I left and I'm starting this vacation at 242 lbs. — down 87.

Commentary

Imagine! I was eagerly anticipating all of the physical activities I'd avoided for years. I was facing challenges – I knew that. But I also knew that I would be focusing on the rewards of losing fat and building muscle — energy and stamina and enjoying that my body could do so much more. I was ready for the great adventure!

👍*FNM*

8/23/04: My New Life, day 153

Today, on the five-month anniversary of my surgery, I did something I never dreamt I'd be able to do. I hiked up Connecticut's highest peak, Bear Mountain, elevation 2330 ft.!

Each day my activity level has increased. On the first day we walked a half-mile to the lake for a swim and back. The second day we walked mountain roads for an hour and then went for our swim. By the third day I was ready to tackle Bald Peak. It was work and I was winded at times, but I kept up. That sure felt good.

Bear Mountain was more of a challenge. We hiked through the woods nearby to hook up with the Appalachian Trail. Once we hit the trail, it was pure up. Clambering over rocks and boulders. Wait! Me clambering and climbing? My legs got tired and I had to stop to catch my breath several times. It was hard, but I was doing it. What a feeling of exhilaration! I had hiked, in the full sense of the word, for the first time in my life. I feel an incredible sense of accomplishment and joy.

Commentary

If I were writing a novel, I could not have chosen a more appropriate and symbolic accomplishment than climbing a mountain. Even the name was perfect! My journey over the past five months had been all uphill. I'd encountered rocks and boulders. I'd gotten tired and taken little breaks. As with climbing Bear Mountain, "It was hard, but I was doing it."

You may not climb Bear Mountain — although I recommend it. But you will be doing things you never felt possible. Have faith in yourself, keep going, and then — celebrate your sense of accomplishment and joy.

8/28/04: My New Life, day 158

I've discovered something about my eating habits. I've stayed very active through most of this trip. I haven't thought about food very much and things are easy. The couple of days the weather was bad and we stayed in, reading and relaxing, I wanted to eat all the time. What is it about relaxing and boredom that makes me want to eat? This is something I need to explore and find answers to.

Commentary

I've become more aware of my body. Not like the old me, when being aware meant knowing I was fat and hating myself for being that way. No, now I'm more aware of how my body works.

I don't yet understand why I feel like eating when I'm relaxing or bored, but I'm aware that I tend to do that and I'm determined to be alert to that tendency and stop doing it. And the better I understand the reasons within my body, the better I can control it.

𝒮FNM

8/31/04: My New Life, day 161

My vacation is over. I walked, hiked, swam, and canoed. I did it all. I no longer feel like I have to sit on the sidelines. That is an incredible feeling! And it's only going to get easier as I continue to lose. When I arrived home, I found that I'd lost 7 lbs. during my vacation, a feat never before accomplished. I've completely changed my concept of vacation.

Commentary

Read the third and fourth sentences again: "I did it all. I no longer feel like I have to sit on the sidelines." You can probably imagine how I felt; you really don't need me to tell you that the feeling was incredible.

You've imagined such feelings, I'm sure — being able to participate fully in physical activities with members of your family and with friends, not sitting on the sidelines of life. And, like me, you'll be able to stop imagining and start actually experiencing those feelings.

𝒮FNM

Wrap-Up

During rapid weight loss our body's hormones can get out of balance. Many hormones are stored in fat cells. As we shrink these fat cells, they release the hormones they've been storing. The result is that we have periods of time with hormonal imbalance. This imbalance can affect our moods and emotions. If you are aware of this, you can be better prepared to deal with it.

In the past most of us have used food to deal with our mood swings and emotional ups and downs. We go to foods that are high in carbohydrates because they will quickly release insulin into our system, the insulin raises serotonin levels in our brain, and the serotonin calms us down and makes us happy.

I'm working on recognizing my emotions and not feeling that I have to immediately hide them or mask them if I judge them to be "bad" emotions. We can allow ourselves to experience the emotions and, if we choose to eat, go for foods that will release insulin slowly and give us sustained energy and feelings of well-being that last. And those are feelings that can help us be fat no more.

 FNM

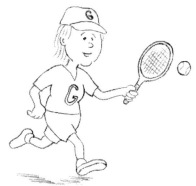

Chapter 9. Sweet Stuff
and Other Cravings

9/1/04: My New Life, day 162

Today I was thinking about my sweets cravings that used to consume me. I haven't had any of those cravings so far, which is a wonderful thing to be free from. I'm tempted from time to time but I don't crave sweets. I think that's because I've eliminated them completely. I was thinking about my vacation last month and how my friends made home-made bread and cookies several times. The smells were hard to get away from in our little cabin and I wanted to join in the baking and the eating like I always have in the past. Those cookies looked so good. My decision to stay away from sweets and sugar completely — not even a little taste — was put to the test.

Commentary

Many people, if they're lucky, lose their craving for certain foods they couldn't resist before, like sweets. Sometimes you lose the physical/physiological craving, but mentally miss the food and want to have it — there's a difference.

This is especially true for gastric bypass patients, since their whole digestive system has been changed. Most cravings return somewhere after six months, but hopefully by this time you've made many of the lifestyle changes that will help you deal better with the cravings.

👍*FNM*

9/1/04, continued

Some people can get away with having a little sugar here and there. I might not even "dump" on sugar like many do after the surgery, but I don't even want to find out. I know that a little taste, for me, can easily lead to much more. I look on sugar the same way an alcoholic needs to consider one drink. I managed to walk away this time.

Commentary

I explained "dumping syndrome" in Chapter 1, but I want to remind you that it's one of the side effects unique to gastric bypass surgery. It's not among the effects of gastric banding, since banding does not alter the digestive system.

Not everyone has "dumping syndrome." Some people can tolerate a little sugar, others can tolerate any amount of sugar, and many of us "dump" on just the smallest amounts of sugar. You don't know which you are. Do you want to find out? I don't. I'm going on the assumption it will make me very sick, so I stay away from sugar. I consider that one of the advantages of this surgery.

FNM

9/7/20: My New Life, day 168

They changed the rules! Last night at our support group meeting, we went over a document called The Rules of the Pouch, written by E.E. Mason, bariatric surgery pioneer. It outlines the rules that post-op patients must follow to be successful, many of which I've covered here. But what many people don't know is that some of the rules change significantly around the six-month mark. The pouch has healed by this time, hunger is back, and there have to be new strategies to continue to shed the pounds and maintain the weight loss.

No more 45-minute meals. I must eat a little faster so the pouch doesn't have time to begin emptying before I finish eating. Meals are a quick 15-20 minutes, still chewing carefully, but not mashing my food to a watery pulp anymore. I want my meal to fill and stretch my pouch. In order to retain that satiety, I now wait an hour or more before drinking any liquids. I also must do something called "water load" 15 minutes before eating. Water loading means to drink as much water as fast as I can in a short span of time. This gives me a full feeling before I even start eating, so I eat less.

These new rules came at the perfect time. I was starting to feel hungry much of the time and it was becoming a struggle to keep from snacking more often. This worried me. Was I going to fail at this? Was it going to become just like any other diet — a constant struggle to stop myself from eating? I read these rules before the surgery, but had forgotten that they changed as your body changed. It's a good thing many people have gone before me. The surgeons and their staff have learned much over the years about how the tools will help us remain successful.

Commentary

The Rules of the Pouch are one of the most important tools for weight-loss surgery patients. (These rules can be found at the back of this book.) Some of the rules apply only to gastric bypass surgery patients. But gastric banding patients find that they can successfully apply many of these rules to their new way of eating also. (Again, they do not have to be concerned about dumping, although they should still avoid sugar.)

Do you have a copy of the rules posted prominently somewhere in your house? Maybe there are a few rules you have a tendency to forget about and skip over in your daily life. You might want to get some brightly colored index cards and write out one rule per card — especially the ones you forget easily. Where could you tape those cards to remind yourself every day about the importance of those rules? Reminders are good things, especially for those of us who find the old brain can't hold as much information as it used to.

👍 *FNM*

10/12/04: My New Life, day 203

Most people don't consider chairs dangerous or worrisome. Not so for a very large person. I have spent a good portion of my life worrying about chairs. Before I went someplace like a concert or restaurant or on an airplane, I would worry about whether I would fit in the chairs. Did the restaurant have booths that would be too narrow or would I be intruding into the space of the person I was seated next to on the airplane? I refused to ask for seatbelt extenders because I felt ashamed. I flew with the seatbelt tucked around me, but not closed. Not the smartest thing I've ever done!

Once I went to a Jenny Craig Weight Loss office to register for their program. When I sat down on the chair they offered, it broke! The humiliation was enough to send me scurrying out of that place. Afterward, I often wondered whether they rigged it that way to encourage clients to sign up for their program immediately.

Today I am FREE from "chairaphobia." I no longer need to worry about the size of the chairs ahead of time. I know that I'll fit. On my vacation, when I flew, it was the most satisfying feeling to sit down, easily buckle my seatbelt, turn to my seat-mate, and carry on a conversation, knowing he hadn't groaned inwardly when "the fat lady" took the seat next to him.

There are so many little things like this in my life that have changed for the better already. I wish our world were made to accommodate people of all sizes, shapes, disabilities, and differences. But it isn't. Until it is, I hope my own experience will help me to better understand the challenges others face fitting into our often unaccommodating world.

Commentary

We often don't realize how our lives have been affected in so many large and small ways by being overweight. The big ones are obvious — like clothes that don't fit, being pointed at by children, feeling uncomfortable in social situations, not being able to do many physical activities without stress or pain, etc. But the smaller ways it intrudes into our lives are pervasive. Sometimes we don't even realize them or don't want to realize them until we start losing the weight and experience the changes for ourselves.

Celebrate those little changes and be proud every day of what you've accomplished. And then keep in mind your memories of feeling embarrassed and uncomfortable — those memories will give you greater strength to resist your cravings.

👍*FNM*

10/23/04: My New Life, day 214

Today is the six-month anniversary of my surgery. I can't believe six months have gone by already. This has been a life-altering experience in every sense of the word. My body, my attitude, and my life have changed immeasurably. I have lost a total of 97 pounds, the size of a young child! I currently weigh 230 pounds instead of 327. In the hips, waist, and bust combined, I am smaller by a total of 34.5 inches and have gone down four sizes.

I have so much energy that there are times I get up and jump or prance around the room just because I feel like it. I've gone from walking a half a mile (on flat terrain) in 20 minutes to briskly walking three miles (adding as many hills as possible) in around 45 minutes. I feel better about my body and don't feel I have to think ahead about whether chairs will fit, if there's too much walking involved, if there are physical activities I can't do, or whether it's someplace I'll feel self-conscious.

The road has not been without bumps so far and will not always be smooth in the future. There are still problems to solve. The surgery has taken care of a large part of the physical problems I faced in losing weight and maintaining the loss, but it doesn't solve the mental and psychological barriers that have kept me from winning this battle before.

I need to find tools and techniques that can help me get past those moments when I'm physically full but continue to feel a need to eat. Those moments when the craving for food, especially carbohydrates, becomes so intense I will do anything to satisfy it, even something that I know can potentially undo all the good and positive I've done. All the determination and good intentions in the world may not be enough to get me past those moments all the time.

What's the solution? I don't know yet, but I'm going to try something called "mindful meditation." I'm starting a class on how to do it and use it this Saturday. I'm arming myself with as many tools as necessary to continue to be fat no more.

Commentary

In later chapters I'll talk more about some of the resources available to us for dealing with many of the mental issues surrounding losing weight and maintaining our weight loss. Remember: this surgery may be a huge step toward solving obesity, but it's not the entire answer. It gives us tools for dealing with many of the physical and physiological barriers to losing weight, but it doesn't address the psychological barriers we have all faced in the past and are bound to face again.

It's important to find techniques and tricks that work for you. Some people brush their teeth more often, because the feel and taste of a fresh mouth can help keep them from snacking. If you can brush your teeth more often, such as immediately after every meal, it's a good habit to acquire. (There may be other benefits as well. People with periodontal disease may be more at risk for heart disease than people without periodontal disease. Periodontal disease also may make it more difficult for people to control their blood sugar. Severe periodontal disease can increase blood sugar, so the body functions with a high blood sugar level for longer periods of time, increasing the risk for diabetic complications.)

👆*FNM*

Wrap-Up

Following weight-loss surgery, foods pass through the smaller stomach without being broken down or digested in the same way. Sugar often moves into the small intestines undigested and the body reacts with symptoms such as clammy skin, heart palpitations, nausea, and diarrhea. Although none of this is life-threatening, it is mighty uncomfortable and something you definitely want to avoid. Not everyone reacts this way — but it's best to play it safe, assume that it's likely, and just avoid sugar completely. For many of us, sugar is like alcohol to an alcoholic — you can't have just a little bit.

Another science break ....

Some sugar is necessary in everyone's diet. Our bodies need sugar to function properly, especially our brains. The food we eat is broken down into glucose (sugar), which our body uses for energy. The better source of sugar is complex carbohydrates, because it takes the body longer to break it down into sugars it can use. Our body can easily handle moderate levels of glucose, using it for energy as we need it. But if we overload our system with too much glucose, our body starts to run out of places to use it and store it, so it sends it to the liver. The liver then converts it to fat and sends it to all the favorite places in our body for fat storage. We all have our special little spots where our body loves to store fat.

When you consume pure sugar, especially large amounts of refined sugar, or any foods high in simple carbohydrates, you feel great — lots of energy. But your body panics at this high level of glucose and a surge of insulin is released so it can lower blood sugar levels. Within a couple hours the glucose levels come crashing down, you feel tired and cranky, and your system craves more sugar and the cycle repeats.

Chronically high carbohydrate consumption leads to chronically high insulin levels. While insulin levels are elevated, your body CANNOT burn fat, you're constantly hungry, and you produce more cholesterol.

Here's what happens when the insulin levels are high.

The liver tries to remove the excess glucose. It converts it to fats — triglycerides and very low density lipoproteins — and secretes it into the bloodstream and breaks down the excess cholesterol into bile acids so it can be eliminated. But if the insulin level remains high, then more cholesterol and triglyceride are synthesized than the body can eliminate.

Excess glucose reacts with proteins in the blood vessel walls and causes inflammation and oxidation, which damages the vessel walls and adjacent nerves. Cholesterol causes similar damage. It's an anti-oxidant, but if the anti-oxidant reserves (vitamins A, C, E, and beta-carotene) are inadequate, the cholesterol will pick up free radicals and become oxidized. The oxidized cholesterol damages certain cells, which become absorbed into the blood vessel walls and start more inflammation and oxidation.

As a result, scar tissue forms, which causes the arteries to harden and become narrower. The consequence is a reduction of the blood supply to body tissues and a rise in blood pressure, increasing our risk of heart disease and diabetes.

So, if you eat a lot of carbohydrates, it's almost impossible to stay on your weight-loss or maintenance program — and you have a greater risk of heart disease and diabetes.

Part of the secret to keeping the cravings at bay is to choose the right kinds of foods for meals and snacks — especially snacks. Foods that raise blood glucose levels slowly and sustain those levels are less likely to start a cycle of craving.

Foods are rated according to how they trigger blood glucose levels. This is called a glycemic index (GI). Each food is given a rating. A food that raises blood glucose levels very quickly is rated high. One that raises blood glucose levels slowly is rated low. Processed and refined starchy foods tend to be high GI. Fresh fruit and vegetables, whole grain, and legumes are low GI. In the back of this book, there's a table showing many of the more common foods and their GI scores.

(Scientists have gone a step further, to develop the concept of glycemic load, a measure of the quality of carbohydrates in a food — glycemic index — and the quantity. The glycemic load of a food is calculated by multiplying the glycemic index by the grams of carbohydrate and dividing the total by 100. If you want to be more scientific about your diet, you should check the glycemic load of your food choices. For most of us, however, knowing the glycemic index is enough.)

Dr. James H. O'Keefe, M.D., director of preventive cardiology at the Mid-America Heart Institute in Kansas City and coauthor of *The Forever Young Diet and Lifestyle*, states that the three biggest obstacles to a healthy diet — for anybody — are high-fructose corn syrup [GI around 85-92] , processed white flour [GI around 70], and refined (white) sugar [GI around 58-65]. "All three of these are sort of predigested food. And because they're so easy to digest, high-fructose corn syrup, processed flour, and refined sugar wash quickly through our systems. They give us too many calories that are too easily consumed and too easily digested. That kicks your body into fat-storage mode. It's another evolutionary adaptation we've developed so that we'd store food in times of caloric abundance. The problem now is that we're always in a time of caloric abundance. So it's no wonder we're getting fat." (Quoted in "The Diet That Conquered the World," by Donovan Webster, *BestLife*, November 2007)

Choosing the right kinds of food and staying away from sugar and other simple carbohydrates (foods with high glycemic indexes) are important steps in making the lifelong changes that will help you become fat no more.

FNM

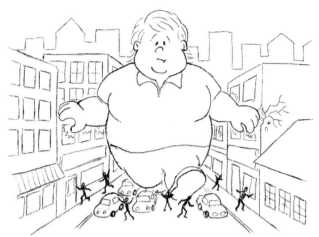

Chapter 10. Freaking Out

10/1/04: My New Life, day 192

100 pounds gone as of today!! I can't quite take it in. When I started this program last March, I hoped for this day — couldn't wait for this day, but deep inside, never thought this day would come. 100 pounds in six months is an incredible accomplishment on any kind of weight-loss program. It's about average for gastric bypass patients. But I don't feel average. I feel like a big winner — or, more correctly, a big loser!

I'm rewarding myself by putting aside money to buy a bike in the spring as soon as the weather starts to turn nice. It feels good to reward myself with something other than food. I think I'm as excited about the bike as I've been about any sweet treat in the past. Can't wait to hit the trails.

Commentary

It's a good idea to come up with ways to reward yourself as you reach different goals and milestones. We are so conditioned to use food as a reward that it's often a struggle to come up with other ideas. Here are a few of my favorites — buy a new piece of clothing I've been drooling over, take the time to have a special outing with a friend I haven't seen in a while (bike rides or walks are great for this), get a massage, buy myself flowers (they just brighten up my day!), take a bubble bath, spend an hour or more in a bookstore, etc.

Here's a little homework for you: write down 10 ways you can reward yourself other than food. Right now, go on! I challenge you to come up with 10.

 FNM

10/12/04: My New Life, day 203

The other day, I saw the father of one of my students for the first time since my surgery. When he came into the room, he stopped and looked at me with a quizzical look on his face and said, "You look different." I smiled, sure he would comment on the weight loss. Then his face brightened in discovery. "I know! You fixed your hair differently." I could only laugh and tell him of course, he was right, because my hair was different. He puffed out his chest and declared proudly, "See, and they say men never notice."

I don't need other people to notice or voice their approval, because I feel good about myself from within.

Commentary

When was the last time you truly felt good about who you are? It's such a relief to not have to seek other people's approval. But it takes time and work and vigilance, because it's easy to slip back into old habits of getting down on yourself. Don't go there! That can lead to that deadly spiral of self-loathing and eating.

👍*FNM*

10/12/04: My New Life, day 203, continued

Thank goodness my hair loss has finally slowed down and wisps of new hair are starting to grow in. Even though I was prepared for this eventuality, it was difficult to watch my hair get thinner and thinner, especially in front. I kept thinking about what cancer patients must go through. That helped keep the hair loss in perspective.

Commentary

Besides, maybe at least some people who know you will think that it's just a new hair style. In fact, you might try wearing your hair differently, maybe only a little more tousled than usual, at least until your hair starts growing back in.

👍*FNM*

10/23/04: My New Life, day 214

The munchies are back! The dreaded munchies are back! Just when I thought I had everything under control and knew all the answers, I get thrown a new challenge. I feel confident that I know what to do to keep the physical hunger at bay, but the hunger that comes from my head is giving me a major pain in the backside.

Commentary

You should always be positive, but you can never assume that your success will continue. There may be setbacks, sometimes dramatic. I was doing so well, weighing 100 pounds less and feeling great, and then — the munchies hit hard. And it's very normal to freak out.

☝*FNM*

10/23/04: My New Life, day 214, continued

I think this is probably the biggest challenge every weight-loss surgery patient faces at one point or another. I know it's a common problem for most people with food issues and I haven't heard of any surefire solutions yet. I'm doing a lot of reading, getting ideas from various books like *Your Erroneous Zones: Step-by-Step Advice for Escaping the Trap of Negative Thinking and Taking Control of Your Life* by Dr. Wayne W. Dyer and *Taming Your Gremlin* by Rick Carson.

Commentary

Remember: the surgery was on our stomachs, not on our heads. It's up to you to search out ways to support your new ways of thinking and doing. That's why you're reading this book — you're not going to expect the surgery to be the cure-all and solve all your problems.

☝*FNM*

10/24/04: My New Life, day 215

Last week, I was feeling out of control. I'd feel hungry, eat something, freak out that I'd eaten something, feel very stressed, and want to eat more. That awful vicious cycle! I was not happy.

I've told family and friends they shouldn't be afraid to eat sweets in front of me. It usually doesn't bother me, until the other day. A friend opened a bag of caramel corn while we were in the car. I couldn't escape the alluring smell. She quickly closed the bag, put it away, and told me it didn't taste that good. But I know a lie when I hear it. The aroma seemed to linger in my car for days. I can't always escape temptation.

This week I'm trying some different tacks. When the cravings hit, I try to drink something first or find an activity to distract myself and hold off eating. Then if I'm still "hungry," I'll have an allowable snack. I'm working hard at not freaking out when I do eat an extra snack. I let it go. I'm also slowing my eating down just a bit again so I can savor my food and feel satisfied physically and mentally when I'm done. I learned those last two tips from my meditation class.

I realize that my worst eating day now isn't as bad as my best eating day in the past. I've got to keep some perspective. I'm still looking for ways to work with my cravings.

Commentary

Are you your worst critic? Do you get into that cycle of getting mad at yourself for giving in to a craving and then, because you're upset, wanting to eat more — or telling yourself, "Oh, I guess I blew it for today. I may as well just not try today and start again tomorrow." Keep your perspective and keep your cool. Being hard on yourself never really worked before, why should it now?

10/26/04: My New Life, day 217

The weight loss has slowed to a crawl. Only eight pounds this month. But it's still crawling in the right direction. I'm down to 219, a grand total of 108 pounds.

Commentary

No matter how slowly I lost weight (and eight pounds a month is not really slow, considering that there have been months when I've gained that much!), my mind has generally lagged behind my body.

I was losing weight faster than my mind could lose the image of my fat body, could get free from "thinking fat." I would be going somewhere and find myself thinking, "Oh, I can't fit in those chairs" or "I can't go through that narrow doorway." And then I'd remember that I was no longer as wide as I'd been for years. I don't need as much space now as for that big body that I've been leaving behind — even as slowly as only eight pounds a month.

11/4/04: My New Life, day 226

Today marks several anniversaries. It's my birthday and one year ago today I made the decision to have bariatric surgery. It was the best decision I've ever made.

For the last couple of years, I didn't look forward to birthdays and getting older. It meant I was getting closer to probable health issues like diabetes and high blood pressure. I felt older and more infirm as walking and standing for any length of time became difficult.

This year I felt like time was going backward and I was getting younger. I am more active, have more energy, and feel like I'm in my 30s instead of my 50s. Maybe by my next birthday, I'll be in my 20s.

Commentary

Not only do you feel younger and more vigorous as you lose the weight, you may also look younger. In a way you are subtracting months and years because, as you lose the weight, you are becoming healthier, putting less stress on your body, and lengthening your life.

11/15/04: My New Life, day 237

I cut up my Lane Bryant and Catherine's credit cards today. Boy, did that feel good! This was another of my major goals — to never have to shop in a large-size store again. I still feel a bit like an intruder when shopping at a regular-size clothing store. I keep waiting for someone to tell me I don't belong there and direct me to the plus-size section.

Commentary

If you're feeling frustrated because you're not losing weight as fast as in earlier months, stroll through the aisles of stores where you used to shop for clothes. Pick up something big and (almost inevitably) drab and hold it up in front of yourself. Think about when you would have bought that item — and then think about what you're able to wear now. A little negative nostalgia may boost your spirits and motivate you to keep on losing.

👍*FNM*

11/18/04: My New Life, day 240

The munchies aren't as much of a problem as they were last month. I think the change from almost no hunger or desire to eat in the first six months, to the normal response to food once again is a hard transition to make. When I talk with other bariatric patients at the seven- to eight-month mark, the problems are similar. Most of us suddenly feel hungry all the time and are haunted by old habits.

I had gotten so used to not caring about food and was sure that would last forever. I felt totally free of food and the mental anguish of wanting, craving, and hunger. To be faced with all of that again is disconcerting at best and down right depressing at times.

I'm learning to adjust and find ways to work with the change. Some successful strategies for me: make sure I only have "good choice" snacks in the house; keep drinking liquids between meals; keep away from simple carbohydrates, since they trigger cravings; meditate; or get busy doing something else. If all that fails, I choose an OK snack, don't get down on myself, and let it go, knowing that I'm doing a great job overall. I'm trying to stay focused on the bigger picture.

👍*FNM*

Wrap-Up

It's never a smooth path to losing or maintaining weight. It's inevitable that you will have difficult days or bad weeks where you find yourself consuming more food than you can burn. Stress, emotional lows, boredom, holidays, physical fatigue, and a myriad number of other reasons can start us down a path we know isn't healthy.

Maybe you're no longer losing weight. Maybe you're even gaining weight. That can happen after six months or after two, three, four, or more years. In fact, maybe you're back to your starting weight. Don't freak out!

It's never too late to get back on track. Do you sometimes feel ready to give up? Don't! You are worth all the effort you've invested in yourself so far — and you're worth all the effort you'll need to continue to put into being fat no more.

The first step is to acknowledge this fact and stop hating and berating yourself, traveling down that old highway spiraling into the place where we've all been before and hoped to never visit again. Forgive yourself and work at changing your mental outlook — before you even think about trying to lose that weight.

Did you ever notice that your thoughts are what create your emotions? Our emotions don't come first; our thoughts do. So the first thing you need to do is change the way you think.

Here are some typical thoughts we might have when we think we've failed:

- "I can't stand it when I lose control of my eating."
- "I'm so stupid to have let things go and gained these 10 pounds."
- "It's so hard to lose those 20 pounds I gained."

Change the thoughts to something more positive, like these:

- "I know I can cut out the carbohydrates for just one day and then it will get easier."
- "I have great information and great tools that I can review and start using again."
- "I lost 150 pounds before. What's a measly 20 pounds? I know I can do it."

Write down a list of positive ways you can start to think about getting your life going the way you want. Consider how you think about your weight, your body, and your efforts to lose. Then decide how you can state those thoughts in a more positive way. You'll immediately feel your mood and emotions start to rise. Tape these positive thoughts some place where you'll see them every day.

One of the books I found helpful on this subject, as I mentioned earlier, is *Taming Your Gremlin* by Rick Carson. This concept is presented in an easy-to-read, upbeat way.

We attract those things in our lives that we think and wish for. We may think we're wishing for something good, but if we always think in the negative, saying what we DON'T want, we're actually attracting the negative. If we always say, "I don't want to be fat," we're attracting being fat. If we say, "I want to be fit and healthy," we attract being fit and healthy. (Yes, in that spirit, the title of this book should be something like *Fit Forever!*)

Don't focus on losing the weight right away, but instead on maintaining where you are. Then review the things you did to lose the weight and what you're doing now that's different. Go over the Rules of the Pouch again. Look at what has worked for you in the past and what you are doing that's working in the present. Continue what's working, reinforce it, and slowly start to reintroduce what was successful in the past. Give yourself little steps that you know you can take successfully.

Write down one step you know you can take today. Maybe it's to do 10 minutes of exercise, or to eat only protein at one meal, or to go for three hours without snacking, or to drink 64 ounces of fluid by the end of the day. Tell someone — a good friend who supports what you're trying to accomplish — about your one step and then report back to that person when you've taken your one step.

The next thing you might want to do is go on a protein-drink fast or limit your food to only protein for a very short period of time. Start with one day. You can manage one day. Don't think past that one day. Then if that goes well and you want to do another day, go ahead. You can do this for up to three days — but any more than that isn't wise, especially without a doctor's supervision. Even after just one day of only protein your body will start to cut back on the cravings.

The other thing you will do on the same day you start your protein fast is engage in some form of physical activity or exercise first thing in the morning, before you do anything else. If you already have an exercise routine in place, that's great: you're one step ahead. If you don't, choose something that you know you can accomplish. If time is an issue, then choose something that doesn't require any preparation time and do it for as much time as you can allow. If that's only 10 minutes, that's OK — it's a start. Try to get in at least 10 minutes every morning and then work up from there.

After your protein fast, slowly add back only carbohydrates low on the glycemic index, so you don't spike your insulin levels and start the cravings again. Remember to take your vitamins and drink your 64-plus ounces of fluids each day.

You should talk about your feelings of failure with other members of your support group. At least some of them will probably understand how you feel through their experiences. You can also benefit from the Web, from the many forums and blogs that focus on weight-loss issues.

A quick search on "weight-loss surgery" and any other terms of interest (e.g., "cravings" or "binges") can lead you to discussions that can help you deal with your issues. Keep in mind that most of the people involved in these discussions are not especially qualified to provide advice. They are talking about their own experiences or what relatives and friends have experienced. But these forums and blogs can serve as part of your social network, to supplement your support groups.

Always be happy and positive about any weight loss you achieve. However little, at least you're moving in the right direction. You'll have some more ups and downs, but keep thinking and feeling positive. You really can be fat no more.

 FNM

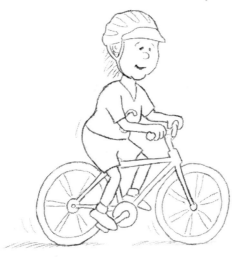

Chapter 11. Have Fun Burning Those Calories!

11/22/04: My New Life, day 244

Thanksgiving and the Christmas holidays are on their way. For me and many people I know, traditionally, these turn out to be big eating frenzies. We're going to my sister's for Thanksgiving. She called yesterday, wanting to know what she could do to make the day easier for me. My family is so thoughtful. She was going to cut out the pumpkin pie so I wouldn't be tempted. I told her to go ahead and serve the usual fare, including the pie. I'll take my low-calorie substitute with me. It's called pumpkin fluff. You mix one box of sugar-free instant vanilla pudding with one and a half cups of skim milk. Then mix in one small can of pumpkin and half of a container of Cool Whip Lite. Add some pumpkin pie spice and extra cinnamon and chill. A half cup of this is about 60 calories, a lot less than pumpkin pie and just as delicious. I'm confident this will see me through the holidays.

Commentary

As I mentioned earlier, in Chapter 5, "Food on the Go," it's essential to plan for social occasions involving food. Your family and friends don't have to do anything special just because of you. Take your provisions — and remember that getting together with family and friends is about socializing, not eating.

11/29/04: My New Life, day 251

I made it through Thanksgiving without any problems. I ate mostly turkey and a tiny bit of everything else except the pie and was content with my pumpkin fluff. My sister worked at keeping the majority of the meal low fat, which was good for everyone. I experienced a feeling of sadness off and on that day. There was a feeling of loss – loss of the freedom to eat everything and as much as I wanted. I knew that the way I was eating was much better for me, but I still missed the food. I was rewarded for my diligence, since I continued to lose this week. My weight loss has now reached a total of 117 pounds. Bring on Christmas!

12/3/04: My New Life, day 255

So now that winter and the cold weather are here, I have to find new ways to get my exercise in. I still have my aerobics and weight training classes, but I can't play tennis and I don't like walking on icy sidewalks or in the extreme cold. The allure of a warm house, fireplace, and cozy couch are difficult to resist. The astounding thing is, my body misses the exercise when I skip. Thought I'd never feel that way. I have a treadmill in the basement (very dusty from years of neglect) and have started using that. I also dug up some old exercise videos. My favorites right now are some old Richard Simmons tapes that combine dance and exercise. Once you get past Richard Simmons' slightly irritating voice, they're fun and very effective.

Commentary

I had used walking as my main source of exercise whenever I was trying to lose weight in the past. A couple weeks before my surgery, I started with short manageable walks (for me that was one or two times around the block) and planned on getting back to it as soon as I was able following the surgery. The surgeons emphasized the importance of getting up and moving for many reasons, including preventing blood clots. Two days after the surgery I walked to the mailbox, the day after that I walked to the end of the block and back, and each day after that I walked a little farther. I set small attainable goals for myself as my strength returned and I healed.

The most important thing was that I had started and established an exercise routine. This would become one of the most important parts of my new lifestyle.

If you're anything like me, you've spent your life avoiding exercise — or at least that part of your life spent overweight. Even as a child, I would much rather sit on the couch reading a book than running around outside like the other kids. Physical exertion was never something that came easy. It was just too hard to move that big body around. The effort was overwhelming. I knew it was good for me — something I needed to do to lose weight and get into better shape. But knowing it was good for me, in fact essential for losing weight, didn't make it any easier.

In this chapter I want to discuss how our bodies burn fat and the benefits of exercise, especially for anyone who has undergone weight-loss surgery. You probably already understand the importance of exercise. The problem is not that you don't have information, but rather that you don't have motivation. I hope to help you find some of that.

What do you want to accomplish with exercise? You might say, to burn more calories and lose weight or, later, maintain your weight loss. Yes, that's definitely something we all want to do. But a better way of looking at it is that, through a regular exercise routine, you can reach a fitness level that allows your body to work with you to burn fat more efficiently so you don't have to feel like you're on a diet the rest of your life.

Our bodies are built to perform incredible tasks. Unfortunately, when you ignore your body for years and don't keep it tuned up, it loses some of those capabilities.

I felt for many years that my body and I were at odds — never seeming to work together. It seemed to fight me whenever I tried to lose weight. It turns out I was right. Because of all the years of neglect, it had temporarily lost the ability to support my efforts.

Our muscles contain enzymes that burn sugar and enzymes that burn fat. Small amounts of sugar (glucose) are stored in every muscle cell and are readily available to use when we need them. So when we begin to exercise, our sugar-burning enzymes go to work first. But the sugar gets used up quickly, because our body doesn't store much sugar. So we run out of energy and want to stop.

The problem is that inactivity decreases our fat-burning enzymes. If these enzymes aren't used, they go away. If they sit there for too long, our bodies break them down and use them in other ways. So when you decide to exercise once a month, the muscles burn sugar only and never get to the point of burning fat.

But don't despair. You can build up those fat-burning enzymes again by exercising consistently.

And here's more reason to exercise. Those fat-burning enzymes don't just abruptly stop as soon as you stop exercising; they continue to work for hours after you're done.

So you can replenish the fat-burning enzymes and increase your metabolism by following an aerobic exercise routine for as little as 15 to 20 minutes a day three times a week. That's only a total of one hour a week! Is it worth it? You bet! Is it going to be easy? Probably not — but it's a lot easier than drastically restricting your calorie intake day after day. Can it be fun? You bet!

FNM

12/13/04: My New Life, day 265

I went to two Christmas parties this past week. I thought I was strong enough to avoid all the tempting goodies — I was wrong. I managed to stay away from the sweets, but the crunchy munchies caught me. The insidious thing about parties is that everything is set out for the purpose of grazing over a long period of time — one of the biggest no-no's for weight-loss surgery patients. You don't realize how much you're eating — the pouch never really fills up.

12/14/04: My New Life, day 266

I've paid for my sins. I gained a pound! This is the first time I've gained in nine months. It's all the fault of those blasted Christmas parties. Next time I'll eat my fill of allowable food, then sip at my sugar-free drink the rest of the time. No more grazing.

Commentary

Once again, it would have been easy — well, no, but possible — to avoid this temptation if I'd brought along provisions. I failed to do so — and I failed to eat right.

FNM

12/15/04: My New Life, day 267

We had our support group meeting last night. We went over strategies for dealing with the holidays — just a few days too late. Oh, well. I did pick up a great idea though. One of the patients who had the surgery 18 months ago and is at her goal told about fasting on protein drinks for a couple days when she feels the need. It helps get the carbs out of her system, which cuts down the cravings. It also helps her jump-start the weight loss when she needs it. It's worth a try.

Commentary

A protein fast is simple — in theory. You eat nothing but lean protein — chicken, fish, eggs, low-fat cheese, and protein drinks.

👍*FNM*

12/22/04: My New Life, day 274

I tried the protein-drink fast for two days this week. It works! It definitely cut my cravings and my appetite down and I lost the pound I'd gained. It wasn't even that difficult.

Other than the one-pound gain, my weight loss has been going very good. I had my thyroid levels checked in November (I have an underactive thyroid) and found they were low. My weight loss had slowed down considerably from September to November. Within a week of increasing the thyroid medication, the pounds started melting off me again. What a relief!

The other thing that has definitely helped kick up the weight loss is a few new activities. I joined a health club and started water aerobics, which I love. I'm also trying out the pilates/yoga class and step aerobics. On the days I don't go to the club, I put on some great rock 'n' roll or jazz CDs and dance around the house, sometimes doing my housecleaning to the music. Anyone looking in my window would think I've gone crazy, but it's fun!

I hate that word "exercise"! The word "exercise" evokes a lifetime of bad feelings, thoughts, and emotions. I tend to think of workouts and gyms and exercise equipment like treadmills and stationary bikes. I prefer the words "physical activity," which can encompass biking, swimming, skating, hiking, walking, dancing, and so much more — things most of us enjoyed doing at one point or another in our lives, mostly as kids. These activities evoke feelings of joy and freedom.

What kinds of activities are going to make my body into the fit fat-burning mechanism it was meant to be? Any activity where you use your muscles to move — as simple as that. The trick is to make that activity into an aerobic exercise.

What makes an activity *aerobic*? That word just means that your exercise is using oxygen, which is necessary to burn fat. Exercise is aerobic when your heart rate is between 60% and 80% of your maximum heart rate.

You can determine your heart rate by wearing a heart monitor or simply finding your pulse on your wrist or neck and counting the beats in six seconds and multiplying by 10. If you do this when you're not active, you get your resting heart rate. Then multiply your resting heart rate by .6 to get the lower limit of your aerobic range and by .8 to get the upper limit.

By the way, exercise is one area where more isn't necessarily better. If you exercise enough to raise your heart rate above 80% or 85% of your maximum, the exercise is *anaerobic* — it's not using oxygen so it's not burning fat.

Keep checking your heart rate, either with the heart monitor or by counting your pulse beats, to make sure you're in your target zone. After a while you don't even need to do that while you're exercising, because you get to know when your body is in that zone.

When you first start moving your body in physical activities after years of being a couch potato, it won't take much to get your heart rate into the aerobic zone. A walk around the block might do it to start with. However, as you become more fit and your cardiovascular system adapts to the increase in exercise, you need to push your intensity up in order to reach that aerobic zone.

Start small. Don't try to become an Olympic athlete overnight. I know it feels good to move your body in the weeks following your surgery, but you have to build up slowly. In the beginning, the best thing you can do is walk. Don't worry about getting aerobic while you're recovering from surgery. But as your body heals, push yourself a little more each day.

As I said, I started with walking to the mailbox and back. Each day I added on a little more — not a big chunk. We sometimes get too eager and go from walking two blocks one day to two miles the next and end up with blisters, sore muscles, or fatigue. Then we wonder why it's so hard to get out there again the next day. Build slowly and then, by six weeks out, with your surgeon's permission, you can move on to trying other forms of physical activity.

Here's something else that's extremely important in getting fit: it isn't always how hard you work at an activity, but the amount of muscle you use. An activity that uses more muscles throughout the body burns more fat at a faster rate than an activity that uses less muscle. If you want to get more benefit from your exercise time, make sure you're using as many muscles as possible.

Let's compare two activities as an example — walking and cross-country skiing. They're both excellent activities, but walking uses only the leg muscles. Cross-country skiing uses practically every muscle you have! The benefits from only 12 minutes of cross-country skiing are comparable to the benefits from 40 minutes of walking.

I don't know about you, but I can't go cross-country skiing every day and even if I could I probably wouldn't want to. I admit it. I'm a cold weather wuss and would rather go walking or biking under warm sunny skies.

If you like to walk, one of the ways you can use more muscles is to use walking poles. Then you engage your upper body muscles and increase your fat-burning output by 20%. You can also turn your walking routine into an aerobic activity is by changing your intensity — walking faster or including hills in your walk.

This is the point to keep in mind when choosing your activities: use more muscles throughout the body and you burn more fat faster.

Probably the most important thing to keep in mind though is to choose activities you enjoy — something you'll want to do again and again, not something you avoid and find every excuse in the world not to do. I can't emphasize this point enough. Just think how great it feels to move your body now that you've been shedding all those pounds. It feels light and free and wants to move. Let it move. Take delight in its movement!

It's taken me a while to find the activities I really enjoy. I've probably tried at least 20 activities in the past three years before I found the ones

I like and am eager to do. My favorites are tennis and biking. But those are hard to do year-round in Wisconsin, so I've had to find substitutes in the winter. Those are harder to find since, as I told you, I'm a cold weather wuss. I'm still searching for the perfect winter activity for me. In the meantime, I do kickboxing, dancing, and spinning — indoor stationary cycling with a leader who takes you through imaginary rides of various terrains and intensities.

I'm lucky. I found that I really enjoy moving my body, being outdoors, and participating in physical activities. Not everyone comes to that naturally or finds the physical drive to push their bodies hard. You don't have to. Your activity program doesn't have to be like anybody else's. It's uniquely yours. It's up to you to find what you will be willing to do consistently. Maybe it isn't much, but it's something that your body will start to crave after a while.

👍*FNM*

12/27/04: My New Life, day 279

I made it through Christmas, had a great time, but didn't go overboard on the food. Christmas Eve in my family is an important time to celebrate all the Polish traditions of the season. That involves many of the foods I grew up with and love, like pierogi, rich and creamy mushroom soup, and poppy seed cake. I filled up on protein and then had one bite of each of my favorites. It was enough to see me through.

Christmas day was harder, with a table laden with cookies and candies. I stayed out of that room. My family is all so supportive and let me choose and make decisions without comments or urging me to have more. They heaped my plate with compliments on how good I looked and that's what got me through.

12/31/04: My New Life, day 283

I did it! I reached my second big goal before the New Year. I am now under 200 pounds — a place I haven't been since I was 25 years old. The weight loss total as of today is 128 pounds in 10 months. That means I lost 11 pounds during the month of December — unheard of.

This has been a remarkable year. I started the year with resolve and hope and I'm ending it with success and joy. In 2005 I look forward to continued success, reaching my next big goal, and trying many new physical activities. Isn't life fantastic!?

Commentary

Establish your exercise program as soon as you're physically able. Why not start as soon as you're home from the hospital and your pain is manageable? This is a great time to start because your motivation is high. You're starting a whole new life!

Find the best time of day for you to walk or do your activity. My best time is first thing in the morning, before the rest of my day gets started and a hundred things distract me. I know that if I leave it for the end of the day when I might have more time, I'm tired and less likely to actually get myself up and going. If you're not a morning person, then consider your lunch break as a possibility. It doesn't take that long to eat our tiny lunches anymore, so there's definitely an opportunity there. But maybe you don't want to get sweaty in the middle of the day, so right after work before you start your evening routine might work best. I know someone who's a night owl and loves to go to the gym at 10 at night and then do her grocery shopping on the way home. Maybe you need to fit most of your activities in on the weekend and then do one additional workout during the week. Do whatever is going to work for you.

As I said before, any physical activity is a good activity as long as you do it consistently and aerobically. Choose what it is you'd like to do and what you are capable of doing. There are so many possibilities — let your imagination go!

You don't have to stick to the prescribed "exercises" everyone else does. Maybe you love to work in the yard or garden. Look at how you can change the way you do it to bring your heart rate up. Go back to the old push mower, dig faster, jog between the garden and the garage with each piece of equipment you need one at a time.

Do you have little kids? Kids bring you endless opportunities for aerobic activity. Put some dance music on and dance with your child. Create an obstacle course of crawling, hopping, slithering, bouncing, etc. Play tag or fetch (you get to do the fetching). Be creative, have fun, and keep your kids fit all at the same time. If your kids are a little older, go for walks, hikes, or bike rides; go skating or swimming; play volleyball, baseball, touch football, soccer, or basketball.

Try different exercise classes and see what you might enjoy. There are neighborhood centers that offer a wide variety of classes. It's more fun to exercise with other people. But if you're a loner, that's OK too. Check out some of the thousands of exercise videos and CDs out there. The used bookstores usually have shelves of various tapes for cheap — everything from pilates and yoga to belly dancing or salsa dancing. Be adventurous!

I find that I do best when I have a variety of activities to choose from. Not only does this keep me from being bored with my fitness routine, but I'm then using different muscle groups. For example, on Tuesdays I do weight training, Thursdays it's a spinning class or biking if the weather is good, Friday it's kickboxing, and the weekend is usually filled with biking, tennis, and walking or hiking.

Walking may be your chosen activity. That's great. Just remember to vary your intensity — especially as you become more fit. Add hills, break into 10- to 30-second jogs every 10 minutes or so, add a 20-lb. backpack. Get a walking partner and challenge each other. Measure your time and distance once a week and see if you can better it the next week. Don't get complacent.

You may have physical limitations that make fitness a bigger challenge. Don't let that stop you. Talk with an exercise physiologist and find out what you can do safely. Very often working out in a pool is going to be easier on your joints or back.

A consistent activity routine is so crucial to your long-term success following weight-loss surgery. If you don't establish a routine and commitment early on it will be much harder to do so later. Get on it right away.

If you've gotten away from your commitment to fitness and are struggling to maintain your weight loss, put back physical activity as a number-one priority. But don't rush back into it, thinking you can start up where you left off. Work your way back up. First thing you want to do is start doing something — anything — consistently again. Don't worry about how much time — you might start with just five to 10 minutes — and don't worry about intensity until you've gotten going again.

If you've been struggling to maintain your weight loss or you've even gained a few pounds back, you don't need to diet (just review your rules of the pouch), you need to raise your fat metabolism. To do that, you need to increase your aerobic energy system, which includes your fat-burning enzymes. Only an aerobic activity program can do that.

As the famous sneaker ad says, "Just do it."

👍 *FNM*

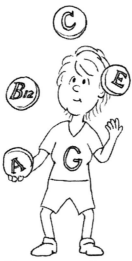

Chapter 12. Remember Your ABCs

1/18/05: My New Life, day 301

I did so well with my food over the holidays that I fell into an old trap. I've been rewarding myself by letting up just a little. Whoa! Not a good idea. I've got to get past this idea that food is a reward. In fact, I need to take some of my attention off food entirely. I do better when I can keep my mind busy, not spend my day planning what I'm going to cook and eat.

Commentary

Losing weight or even simply maintaining our weight can be difficult — and holidays are often the worst time. So, if we do well, we may feel entitled to a reward. That's OK — whatever works to motivate you to keep going and keep getting healthier.

But ... food is a dangerous reward. Not in itself, of course, not in terms of calories or fat. It's dangerous because you're rewarding the new you in terms of the old you. Find other rewards, rewards that support and reinforce your new life. As I've mentioned, clothes can be a good reward — they can make you feel even better about your improving body and, obviously, you need clothes that fit. Or you can buy yourself a new bicycle or new walking shoes, necessities in your new life style.

You don't have to buy something to reward yourself. Maybe luxuriating in a long bath, going dancing, taking time to sit and read, visiting a museum, or other activities are little treats you would enjoy.

And part of that new lifestyle is to keep busy. Most of us go to food for comfort when we're lonely, sad, angry, or bored. So, keeping busy is good — but not so busy that you're completely stressed out. That is definitely not good. Stress can also drive us to food for comfort.

Which feelings are triggers for you? Next time you have an urge to go to the fridge, stop and ask yourself, "What am I feeling right now?" The more you can start to identify your triggers, the more you can avoid them or find different outlets for those feelings.

FNM

1/18/05: My New Life, day 301, continued

So, letting up a little got me in trouble. I gained two pounds this week. My heart sank when I looked at the scale. But I didn't freak out and tell myself I was a failure and a bad person and go eat more — my old way of dealing with it. I just made the decision to go on a two-day protein shake fast again and then cut back and be more careful. This made me realize that some things would never change for me. I would have to be vigilant for the rest of my life. Food and weight were always going to be issues that I couldn't be complacent about, no matter how much weight I lost. It was a reality check.

Commentary

Do you think that gastric surgery resolves all the food issues that have caused you to gain all that weight? You'd be surprised how many people still think the surgery is the answer to all their problems and think they'll never have to watch what they eat again. Sure, it's called weight-loss surgery, but that term does not represent a guarantee, just a good start.

I know there was a point where I was under the illusion that once I had the surgery and lost the weight I'd magically be able to maintain the weight loss just because my stomach was smaller. Wrong. I've got a lifetime of habits and incorrect thinking to change. I'm still working on them.

FNM

1/24/05: My New Life, day 306

I lost the two pounds I gained and am back on track. This is the difference in my life now, I have the tools to deal with the weight and I don't go into despair when things take a temporary turn for the worse. It's temporary.

I can eat almost anything now and the choices sometimes overwhelm me. I make sure I only have healthy food around the house and have even started buying more organic food. Since our systems don't absorb as many of the nutrients as before, I want to make sure that what I'm putting in will do the most to keep me healthy. I have always been religious about taking all the vitamins recommended in our program. In fact, I take an extra B complex for stress, an extra 500 mg of C, omega-3 fatty acid for cell health, acidophilus for digestive health, and a fiber supplement.

Commentary

Many programs differ in what they recommend for vitamin supplements. In my program, with gastric bypass, we are instructed to include in our daily regimen a multivitamin, an extra B complex, 500 mg of B12, 1,000 mg of calcium, and extra iron for certain patients, especially women who are still menstruating. I know that I'm meeting my basic needs with these supplements, but I like to look beyond my basic needs.

There has been a lot of controversy about vitamin supplements over the years. Many traditional health practitioners have felt there was no need for additional supplements except in special cases. But that's changing as more research is being done on the benefits of certain supplements.

Gastric bypass patients definitely fall into the category of "special cases." Remember: when the surgeon made the new connection between our pouch and our small intestines, he or she bypassed a section of the intestines that is partially responsible for absorbing many of the nutrients we get from our food. So we can't count on food alone for the vitamins and minerals we need.

Vitamin deficiencies can cause serious health issues. As an example, a deficiency of B1 can cause an enlarged heart, mental confusion, loss of reflexes, difficulty walking, and even paralysis. Believe me, this can happen; I've seen it. Other deficiencies aren't as serious, but why take any chances?

The following are the specific recommendations of the UW Health Bariatric Surgery Nutrition Program at the University of Wisconsin Hospital, Madison:

After the gastric bypass procedure:

• Chewable multivitamin — two a day
• Calcium — 1,200-1,500 mg daily as calcium citrate
• Vitamin B12 supplement — 500 mcg a day
• Vitamin B-Complex or B-50 — once a day
• Iron — for menstruating women or history of anemia

Iron and calcium must be taken about four hours apart.

After the LAP-BAND® System procedure:

• Chewable multivitamin — one a day
• Calcium — 1,000 mg daily as calcium citrate
• Vitamin B-Complex or B-50 — once a day

Iron and calcium must be taken about four hours apart.

The B vitamins help our bodies deal with stress — physical, mental, and emotional stress.

And the B vitamins are water-soluble: they're broken down by fluids, so if we give our body more than it can use, it just expels the excess. There's no danger of accumulating toxic levels.

I take extra vitamin C because it helps me absorb iron and it strengthens resistance to infections. Vitamin C is also water-soluble. You do have to be careful not to overdo the vitamin C, since it can cause diarrhea if your system isn't used to large doses. If you're going to take extra, build up slowly.

If you have a gastric banding procedure, you don't have to worry about vitamin deficiencies — at least not because of the surgery. However, if you're overweight, there are reasons: you did not eat properly. Now that you have a second chance to eat right, you should know as much as possible about proper nutrition so that you get what your body needs as you reduce the quantity of the food you eat and you eliminate certain foods from your new life.

Omega-3 fatty acids are a nutrient we've been more aware of recently. More information is coming out all the time about the numerous benefits of omega-3.

According to the American Heart Association, omega-3 can be a large factor in continuing cardiovascular health by lowering blood pressure and cholesterol and helping to prevent the buildup of plaque in our blood vessels. Omega-3 has also been shown to have the following benefits:

• It reduces inflammation.

• It alleviates symptoms of depression.

• It helps break up blood clots.

• It helps prevent breast, colon, and prostate cancer.

• It promotes weight loss by lowering insulin levels, which means you are better able to burn stored fat.

• It helps prevent osteoporosis by raising calcium levels.

That's a pretty impressive list of benefits.

Fiber has been found to be a key component of weight loss and overall good health. Earlier in the book we discussed that when our carbohydrates are high in fiber, low on the glycemic index, our digestive system releases blood sugar (glucose) more gradually into the bloodstream and, as a result, the pancreas releases insulin more gradually and the levels are sustained longer.

There are so many other benefits of fiber — from lowering cholesterol to controlling diabetes and lowering the risk of colon cancer. But a very important one for weight-loss surgery patients is that fiber helps prevent constipation.

I've heard so many post-ops complain about constipation. This is a common problem for several reasons. First of all, our diet following surgery consists of mostly protein. Our new stomachs usually don't tolerate raw fruits and vegetables or whole grains. So we're not getting the fiber we need to keep things moving along through the digestive tract. Drinking the required liquids can often solve this problem, but not always. Sometimes a fiber supplement will help. Just make sure you drink LOTS of liquid with any kind of fiber supplement or you'll be in even more trouble. If you take fiber supplements without adequate fluids, they may cause choking.

As your eating changes and you can tolerate more foods, the best source of fiber is fresh vegetables and fresh fruit. We're still going light on the carbohydrates and not adding a lot of grains, so it's even more important that when you add them, you're adding whole grains. Once again, whole grains have more fiber, raise our blood sugar levels more gradually, and provide more nutrients.

I remember when a radical group of health food fanatics in the '60s started preaching that white sugar and white flour were "death." They were dismissed as "crazies" — but they were just in the forefront of what we know now.

When carbohydrates are refined, the process removes fiber, healthy oils, vitamins, and minerals, transforming complex carbohydrates into simple carbohydrates.

Refined flour is almost pure starch, with no protein. It breaks down rapidly into sugars. When the digested starch enters the small intestine, the result is a surge of sugar into the bloodstream. To control this surge, the body rapidly produces insulin and the liver works harder to process the excess. The body can be too efficient, lowering the sugar level in the bloodstream too far, which means that we become low on energy. The roller coaster of blood sugar levels can stress the body's ability to control blood sugar. The result can be diabetes. Refined sugar is even worse than refined flour: it requires no digestion to cause a dangerous surge of sugar into the bloodstream.

1/27/05: My New Life, day 309

I started seeing a therapist this month. My eating has always revolved around emotional issues. Food had been my way of avoiding. So now I have these emotions staring me in the face, demanding attention, and I can no longer ignore them. What do I do with them? I especially need help with what I've always considered the negative emotions — sadness, anger, and fear. Hopefully a professional will help me choose ways other than eating to react to what life throws at me.

Commentary

As I mentioned earlier in this chapter, we can't expect gastric surgery to resolve our food issues. Also, losing weight is not just a matter of mind over body. Yes, that's important, of course. But what's in our heads and our hearts can determine what goes into our bodies. Until we can break or at least control that link, our bodies will remain vulnerable to our emotions.

1/30/05: My New Life, day 312

Being more vigilant has paid off. I lost two more pounds this week. Six pounds this month, so I have now lost a total of 135 pounds! People keep saying to me lately, "You're so small!" Boy, does that make me feel good!

I have never been small or thought of myself as small. In fact "small" has never been a word that anyone has ever used paired up with my name before. I have to continually readjust how I think of myself now. My mind and perceptions haven't quite caught up to my body yet, but I've got plenty of time — the rest of my life.

Commentary

As you lose weight and as you live more actively, try to pause from time to time and think of how a friend might describe you at this moment to someone who's never met you. What adjectives and adverbs would be most accurate? As you improve your body and your life, work at improving your self-image.

2/7/05: My New Life, day 321

I always believed that my life was great except for my weight problem. I thought that if I could lose the weight, all my problems would be solved and everything would be wonderful. Wrong.

Yes, the weight loss certainly has made my life better in so many significant ways, but it didn't magically make everything better. It had become my catch-all excuse for anything that went wrong in my life. Time to find a new excuse? I guess not.

Commentary

The emotional changes and ups and downs that follow this surgery can sometimes be overwhelming. I was aware of the fact that I'd be facing psychological and emotional challenges, but nothing quite prepared me for what I alone would be facing, the reality of my personal challenges. Everyone is different and no one can completely predict what will trigger a stressful reaction for you. I'll talk more about this issue in a later chapter.

2/12/05: My New Life, day 326

Haven't lost anything in two weeks, but I haven't gained either. Someone asked me today if I was almost at my goal. My response was "Of course not! I'm nowhere near my goal!" Then they asked how many more pounds I wanted to lose and I said "35 more."

Suddenly it hit me — that isn't that much. It's something I can definitely achieve. It may take me a while yet, especially now that the weight loss has slowed, but it isn't something in the far distant future anymore. I had gotten so used to talking about losing more than a hundred pounds. 35 is a small number.

Wrap-Up

Weight-loss surgery can help us control how much we eat, but it's up to us to make wise choices about what we eat. Our systems are no longer as efficient at extracting the nutrients from our food, so it's even more important we choose foods that are highly nutritious. We should primarily be eating lean proteins, vegetables, fruits, and whole grains. We should be avoiding sugar and products made with refined flour.

It's up to you to control your environment as much as you can. What kinds of food do you have around your house? Are they foods that will enable you to lose the weight you need to lose and then maintain your target weight? Or are they foods that you find hard to resist and that will lead you back into your old patterns of eating?

Are you providing and preparing food for others? Do you keep snacks around for kids and/or a partner? Consider this a time to make changes in their eating habits also.

Do you want your children to have the same weight struggles and issues that you've had? Here's a chance to help get them on a path to healthier eating. You may not be able to change everything overnight if you don't want to provoke a major rebellion, but you can make changes gradually. Choose snacks made from whole grains. Add more fruit to their choices. Move away from sugary sodas and introduce alternatives like carbonated waters flavored with natural juices.

When preparing meals, there's no need to make two different meals — one for you and one for them. There are good cookbooks out there that offer flavorful recipes that will meet your needs and satisfy your family's taste buds. In Chapter 3 I listed four cookbooks that can help you. Also, many of your favorite recipes can be made healthier. For example, *Culinary Classics: Essentials of Cooking for the Gastric Bypass Patient* by David Fouts contains some 120 recipes that your family can enjoy with you. There are dozens of Web sites that not only offer good low-carb recipes, but convert many of our old favorites into healthier choices. (The Resources section at the back of this book lists the cookbooks that I've mentioned and some good Web sites.) You can also share recipes with the other members of your support groups. As I've mentioned earlier, that's one of the things we do in my support groups.

Because our systems cannot process foods in the same way and thus deprive us of some of the nutrients, it is extremely important to always take the vitamins recommended by our doctors. There are many options out there for bariatric patients, including specially formulated vitamins, which their promoters claim to be easier to absorb. Your doctor can advise you on the vitamins that will work best for you.

Possible Nutrient Concerns After Bariatric Surgery

(Courtesy of UW Health Bariatric Surgery Program,
© 2008 University of Wisconsin Hospitals and Clinics Authority)

Nutrient: Vitamin B12

Signs and Symptoms of Deficiency:

Tongue: Smooth, shiny, swollen, cracks, red, sore
Blood: Macrocytic anemia (fatigue, weakness)
Skin: Hypersensitivity, hyperpigmentation, pallor
Nervous System: Peripheral neuropathy (tingling in hands and/or feet), ataxia (uncoordinated)

Tests to Indicate Status:

Blood draw for:
— low B12 level
— low mean cell volume
— high serum methylmalonic acid

Preventive Treatment:

500-100 mcg sublingual (under the tongue) Vitamin B12 or monthly intramuscular injections of Vitamin B12 (from your primary care physician, not available over the counter)

Nutrient: Folate

Signs and Symptoms of Deficiency:

Blood: Macrocytic anemia (fatigue, weakness)
Tongue: Smooth, shiny, swollen, red, cracks
Nervous System: Fatigue, depression, confusion
GI Tract: Diarrhea
Immune System: Suppression (increased infections)

Tests to Indicate Status:

Blood draw for:
— low serum folate
— high mean cell volume

Preventive Treatment:

B complex or B-50 with folate

Nutrient: Thiamine

Signs and Symptoms of Deficiency:

Nervous System: Mental confusion, irritation, dizziness, peripheral
paralysis, nystygmus (darting eyes), foot drop
Muscles: Weakness, wasting, painful or numb calf

Tests to Indicate Status:

Blood draw for:
— low whole blood thiamine

Preventive Treatment:

B complex or B-50 with thiamine

Nutrient: Iron

Signs and Symptoms of Deficiency:

Blood: Microcytic hypochromic anemia (fatigue, weakness)
Tongue: Smooth, shiny, red, painful, may be pale in later stages
Other: Pallor, irritability, dizziness, shortness of breath, brittle or
spooning nails, pale lining of eyes

Tests to Indicate Status:

Blood draw for:
— low serum iron (Fe)
— low hemoglobin/hematocrit
— low mean cell volume
— low serum ferritin
— high TIBC (total iron binding capacity)

Preventive Treatment:

Complete multivitamin with iron
Additional iron supplement if menstruating heavily or history of anemia

Nutrient: Calcium / Vitamin D

Signs and Symptoms of Deficiency:

Bone: Osteoporosis and ostoemalacia (softening of bones, bone fractures, bone pain)

Tests to Indicate Status:

Low bone density
Blood draw for:
— high PTH (parathyroid hormone)

Preventive Treatment:

1200-1500 mg calcium citrate with Vitamin D
Additional 800 IU vitamin D if previously vitamin D deficient

Notes

Supplements listed are available over the counter.

Toxicity (too much) with B vitamins is rare because the kidneys filter out unneeded B vitamins. Niacin, folate, and vitamin B6 can have toxicity symptoms with intake of very high doses (over 75 mg, 500 mg, and 500 mg, respectively), but usually only with prolonged intake. There are no toxicity concerns with high blood levels of vitamin B12 or thiamine.

Very high levels of vitamin D (>80) can lead to calcium deposits around the body. This usually only happens with years of high vitamin D levels and with inappropriate long-term treatment of 50,000 IU of vitamin D.

Glossary

Calcium — This test measures the concentration of total and ionized calcium in the blood to reflect parathyroid function and calcium metabolism.

Vitamin B1 (aka thiamine) — This vitamin helps the body cells convert carbohydrates into energy. It is also essential for the functioning of the heart, muscles, and nervous system.

Vitamin B12 — This vitamin is important for normal nerve activity and cell division. It is an important measurement in the determination of anemia.

Vitamin D — This vitamin is required for absorption of calcium. It regulates blood calcium levels by taking calcium from bones if not available in the diet.

Parathyroid hormone (PTH) — This hormone is produced in the parathyroid gland and is important in the regulation of calcium concentration. A high value may mean that the body is stealing calcium from the bones even though calcium levels may be normal.

Hematocrit — This test indirectly measures the red blood cell mass. The result is the percent of red blood cells in whole blood. It is an important measurement in the determination of anemia.

Ferritin — This test reflects the body iron stores and is a good indication of iron storage status. The test is used to diagnose deficiency or overload.

TSH — Thyroid stimulating hormone measurement is the single most sensitive test for primary hypothyroidism.

Wrap-Up

As I've mentioned earlier, I'm very conscientious about taking all my vitamins and have enjoyed excellent health over the past four years. Yet, twice when I've gone in for my yearly follow-up with my surgeon, my blood tests have shown that I was low in a couple nutrients. And that has happened even when I take all my vitamins and eat healthy!

What about all the bariatric patients out there who never take their vitamins? Are they putting themselves at major risk for health issues in the future? It may not be obvious now in the short term, but what about the long term?

When we make the decision to take the big step of weight-loss surgery, it's to make our lives better. Good health is part of a better life. Personally, I know I want to be in good health so I can enjoy my new body and my new life. Healthy eating and taking the prescribed vitamins are essential for my new life and my new body — which I am determined will be fat no more.

FNM

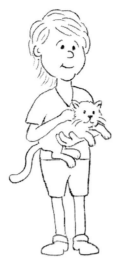

Chapter 13. Under the Knife Again

4/4/05: My New Life, day 377

One year after my gastric bypass surgery, I met with Dr. Gould for my one-year checkup. Drs. Garren and Gould chart everyone's progress at one year and my 155-pound weight loss coincides almost exactly with the average. So my weight loss is neither exceptional nor slow. But average is completely satisfactory to me. Dr. Gould also suggested I move ahead with checking into plastic surgery to get rid of the excess skin.

Commentary

Have you considered plastic surgery? Many programs suggest that if you're thinking of plastic surgery you wait until sometime after the first year, when you've lost all the weight you want to lose or think you're going to lose and have remained at a stable weight for at least six months. It can sometimes be a long process to get scheduled for plastic surgery and you may want to start well ahead of when you want it done.

It's a downside of success in losing weight: we may shrink our bodies, but our skin tends not to shrink. So we usually have lots of skin that we no longer need, especially on our bellies, thighs, breasts, and upper arms. Exercise is not very effective in shrinking skin. It may shrink a little over time, but don't expect miracles.

4/26/05: My New Life, day 399

I have an appointment tomorrow with Dr. Karol Gutowski, a plastic surgeon who is highly recommended for bariatric patients. I want to get rid of this extra skin. I have constant rashes and infections in the folds of the skin. I'm on oral medication and two topical medications for the rashes and it's still a problem that's only going to get worse as the weather gets hotter. Yet, I don't feel ready to move ahead because I don't think of myself as "done" or thin yet. But will I ever feel "done" or thin? If I wait for that, I could be waiting forever. It's time to at least check it out.

4/27/05: My New Life, day 400

I nearly kissed Dr. Gutowski when he told me not to bother trying to lose more weight at this point! Most of my excess weight is now sitting in my midsection and legs. He said he would handle the midsection with surgery. He also said you can't "spot lose" in the legs and if I want those smaller I'd have to have it removed surgically as well. If I get the OK from the insurance company, I will have a circumferential abdominoplasty. This means that the incision will run all the way around and include removal of excess skin from front and back. He will also do what's called a body contour, which means removing any excess fat and tightening the skin across the stomach, hips, and buttocks. It's amazing what they can do.

We also discussed a breast reduction and lift in the future. I've had back problems all my life, which have continued. Being large on top has its drawbacks. Plus now, the sag is astonishing. I read one woman on the discussion boards describe her breasts as two large tube socks with sand in the toes. I think that appropriately describes mine, except I have more sand.

Commentary

It's important to document health problems that are due to the excess skin. Insurance companies vary greatly on whether they'll cover surgery to remove excess skin after a large weight loss.

If they cover the surgery, it's only because it is deemed a medical necessity. Severe rashes that won't clear up with standard treatment often come under the category of medical necessity. It's important that you seek medical treatment for this condition so you can prove you've gone through standard treatments. It's also a good idea to take pictures of times when your rash is severe so you have even more proof to document your claims if needed.

Sometimes you need to be aggressive with insurance companies and not take "no" for an answer. There is usually an appeals process you can go through. You may have used that process to get your weight-loss surgery covered — and you may have to use it again or any other tricks you've learned for dealing with your insurance company.

Tummy tucks and breast reductions are the most commonly covered — if covered at all. Breast enhancement, thighs, and arms are usually not covered; if you want to have any of these procedures done, you'll probably be paying for them yourself. Check with your insurance company to see if they cover any plastic surgery.

👍*FNM*

5/20/05: My New Life, day 423

I've gotten the go-ahead from the insurance! Surgery is scheduled for July 14. I'm not jumping for joy at the thought of more surgery, but I'm focusing on the outcome.

6/5/05: My New Life, day 439

My weight had pretty much stabilized over the past three months with an occasional pound lost. That changed over the month of June. I've found a new physical activity I love. I started bicycling at the end of May and I've lost 10 pounds this past month! What a nice surprise. I've been riding the bike trails around Madison and I'm up to 15 to 30 miles per outing. I also went kayaking up at my sister's for the first time. It was a beautiful experience.

The interesting thing is that I've been eating a little more. I'm sure it's the combination of the increased exercise, plus I believe my overall metabolism has increased. My weight loss is now at minus 165 pounds. The surgery will take off an estimated 10 pounds. That will put me exactly where I had hoped to be someday. I guess "someday" is about here.

Commentary

Adding a new physical activity or changing the way you do your current activities can often jump-start your weight loss again. Our bodies adjust to the level of activity we're doing. Also, as we become more fit and our body is more efficient at expending energy, we aren't reaching our target heart rate zone with the same level of activity. So, push a little harder, try something new, lengthen your workout time, add interval training, or re-evaluate and fine-tune what you're doing currently.

You may not be familiar with the concept of interval training. It's generally defined as repetitions of high-intensity activity followed by periods of low activity or even rest. Many fitness experts believe that interval training is more effective at helping reduce fat than training at a moderate intensity for the same length of time.

👍*FNM*

7/24/05: My New Life, day 488

I had my abdominoplasty on July 14. Before the surgery, I read on the discussion boards that some people had all their plastic surgeries done at one time — stomach, legs, arms, and breasts. Wow! I'm glad I didn't do that. I felt that I had enough to deal with just having the one procedure.

I had asked Dr. Gutowski if it was better to have them all done at once or not. He said that it's too much trauma for our bodies to go through that amount of surgery at once. He wouldn't recommend it and he wouldn't do it. I was glad to hear that.

My surgery went well, but I have a large incision to care for. There's not as much pain as I expected because much of the area around the incision is numb, but it's extremely uncomfortable. This surgery doesn't mess with your internal organs, so most of the pain is on the surface.

I had to sleep sitting up in a recliner for the first week. I'm back to sleeping in bed, but I don't sleep for very long periods of time as I have to keep shifting my position. I have to wear a binder day and night. It's almost like a girdle that you pull around you and close with Velcro®. It's not the most comfortable, but holds everything together. I know it's not possible, but I have this terrible image of my whole body just coming apart in two halves if I don't wear the binder to hold it together!

7/29/05: My New Life, day 493

I developed an infection where the two incisions meet — the one that goes all the way around my body and the one that makes a T with the incision that comes down from my belly button in the front. I had read that it's not uncommon for weight-loss surgery patients to develop infections following plastic surgery. I'm on antibiotics, but the infection has really wiped me out physically. It feels like a major assault on my entire body — and I guess it is.

Commentary

There are risks with any kind of surgery. One of those risks is infection at the incision site. That's one of the big advantages of laparoscopic surgery — much less risk of infections. But with plastic surgery this risk can't be avoided — especially when the incision covers such a large area as in an abdominoplasty.

It's important to do some research to find a competent plastic surgeon with an excellent reputation who has experience working with weight-loss surgery patients. Your bariatric surgeon can often refer you to someone local that he or she feels confident will do a great job. But never hesitate to ask around, interview more than one surgeon, ask to see before-and-after pictures of each surgeon's previous patients, and carefully choose someone you know you can trust.

👍*FNM*

8/15/05: My New Life, day 510

It's taking forever to recover from the abdominoplasty. The infection I developed took a lot out of me and I'm not bouncing back like I expected. I'm not supposed to exercise vigorously for six weeks, but I'm itching to get out and do something. I've been walking one to two miles most days and today I decided to take my bicycle out for an easy ride around the neighborhood. It wiped me out, but it felt good to ride again.

8/19/04: My New Life, day 514

I'm thin! I couldn't say that before — the words would get stuck in my throat. I felt like a fraud. Who was I fooling, trying to pass myself off as thin? I constantly marvel at the head games that accompany this amount of weight loss. My mind has trouble making the adjustments as fast as my body has. After all, I've spent over 40 years thinking of myself as fat, too big, overweight, and many other not too flattering adjectives.

What really made the difference for me was getting rid of the belly. I knew it was mostly excess skin, but having it there kept my negative perceptions focused on that part of myself. It's the part of my body that I always thought of as too big. With that gone, I can begin to see myself as a thin person. I can now say it without blushing or choking. I'm thin!

Commentary

As I recommended in the previous chapter, it's good to pause from time to time as you're losing weight and becoming more active and think about how friends might describe you now. As you work to free your body from that excess weight, work to free your mind from negative images that are weighing you down psychologically.

FNM

Wrap-Up

To have plastic surgery or not — that's a big question most weight-loss surgery patients face at some point in their journey of change. For some the question revolves around body image. Are you satisfied with the body you have following your weight loss? Do you feel healthy and fit and that's your focus? Maybe you feel that the quest for "the perfect body" is not what your life is about. Or you don't have any health issues related to excess skin. Maybe you're one of the lucky ones who have very little excess skin. Then plastic surgery is not a priority.

Maybe you don't want to go through another surgery. Any surgery is a risk, although the risks are less with plastic surgery than with major surgery. Surgeries also take time out of our lives — time away from jobs and families and other priorities. And for me, it meant being unable to exercise vigorously for six weeks. That's become one of my "other priorities."

Maybe you're concerned about finances and whether or not the surgery would be covered by your insurance company. Few plastic surgeries are covered; even when they are, there's usually a deductible or co-pay to fork out. You can figure that most procedures are going to start somewhere over $5,000. You might choose the one area in your body that makes you the most unhappy and start a plastic surgery fund.

Again the question comes up — how happy are you with the body you have when you reach your target weight? Give that question some time and thought as you move into the maintenance phase of your journey. Unless there is an overwhelming medical reason to move ahead right away, it's good to give your body time to adjust. Your body may still be changing and adjusting for another year or more after you reach your goal or the point where you've stopped losing weight.

If you're thinking of going ahead with plastic surgery, what can you expect? Consult with a plastic surgeon well ahead of when you'll be scheduling your surgery. Find out if you're ready for surgery, what procedures the surgeon would suggest, what the estimated recovery time is, what the risks and possible complications are, and what you can do to prepare for the surgery. Find out all the answers to your insurance or payment questions.

Everyone's experiences with plastic surgery are different. Pain, recovery time, complications, and overall satisfaction can vary greatly. Check out some of the message boards; ask questions, learn about other people's experiences, and find out about any potential problems. I spent a good deal of time on the plastic surgery message board at ObesityHelp.com before I made a decision.

Plastic surgery leaves scars. There are treatments for scars, ranging from rubbing on oils for months after to applying specially formulated ointments or patches for a period of time. Scars can lighten and, over time, sometimes become almost indiscernible. If you're having your arms done so you can wear sleeveless shirts or your legs done so you look good in short shorts, you may not be completely satisfied with the results.

Plastic surgery can be that final step to feeling good about the body you have. It may not be perfect, but you can be proud of the steps you've taken, the changes you've implemented, and your determination to be fat no more.

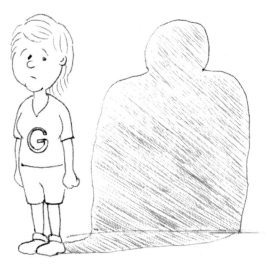

Chapter 14. Problems with Your Body May Be in Your Head

10/20/05: My New Life, day 576

One of my biggest fears when embarking on this journey was that I would change from a "fat jolly" person to a "skinny bitch." I've spent my life being happy, upbeat, and nice. I felt I had to be extra nice so people would like me. I was so afraid they would judge me by my looks, so I would overcompensate with personality.

My husband told me when we had our second date that I was the nicest person he ever met. Recently he told me I'm not as nice as I used to be. Uh-oh! Am I turning into a skinny bitch? He said I went through a bitchy stage as my hormones adjusted, but overall it isn't that bad. Thank goodness!

I've noticed that I'm not as concerned with making everyone like me. My attitude has become a gentle "you can take me or leave me as I am." I think that's a much healthier attitude. I did check with several friends, though, and they agree that I'm still a nice person — a little more assertive, but still nice.

Commentary

Sometimes when we're losing weight we seem or act "less jolly" because we no longer feel a need to make everybody like us. That seems logical, as an effect of feeling better about ourselves, building our self-esteem.

Sometimes we're less cheerful because we're reacting to the new restrictions and requirements. That's completely normal — and even to be expected.

Sometimes the situation is more serious. Sometimes people who've undergone weight-loss surgery feel down, even depressed. If that's the case for you, it may be in part because your expectations for surgery were too high. Again, surgery is not a cure-all; it just gives us a fighting chance to lose weight and live healthier, happier lives. There are no guarantees.

If your surgery was gastric bypass, the cause of the depression could also be physiological. You no longer have the natural functions of the duodenum and the upper portion of the jejunum. Since the body cannot absorb vitamins (especially B12) and minerals and fats, you may be suffering from deficiencies that could be at least partially the cause of your depression. We know that gastric surgery works, but the experts do not agree on the reasons for that success. It seems smart, then, to continue getting check-ups to make sure you're giving your new body the nutrition it needs to function properly. Make sure that you're getting enough of the vitamins, minerals, amino acids, and other things your body needs, from your food and from supplements.

People can also feel down because they lack a social network. It's extremely important to attend support group meetings or at least keep in contact with the members of your support group. We all go through periods when we feel down, when we feel frustrated. It can help a lot to talk with others who have gone through similar experiences.

10/23/05: My New Life, day 579

This morning I found myself dancing around the kitchen. I felt such a lightness of being and it was a joy to be able to express that with my body.

Commentary

It's such a wondrous joy to feel this way about my body! This feeling reminds me of some words of wisdom attributed to several people: "When you finally allow yourself to trust joy and embrace it, you will find that you dance with everything."

10/23/05: My New Life, day 579

I think I need to get a second job to pay for all the lovely clothes I want to buy all the time. I have to keep reminding myself that just because something fits and looks good doesn't mean I have to buy it.

Commentary

Am I addicted to shopping now? No, I like clothes a lot and spend more on clothes now than I ever did, but it's not an addiction. I recognize addiction because I know I have an addiction to sugar and food in general. It's something I've come to accept and continue to work on. But I have seen, read about, and heard about people who, following weight-loss surgery, find that their addictive personalities are developing behaviors in other areas.

Maybe you saw the Oprah Winfrey show about replacement addictions. Maybe you've read about them. It's been estimated that 30% of gastric surgery patients develop a new addiction to replace their addiction to food. Most become addicted to alcohol, some to sex, some to medications such as Vicodin, some to compulsive shopping, some to gambling, some to smoking ....

What is "addiction"? We use that word a lot and sometimes inaccurately. It's a matter of doing something to excess and not being in control.

Maybe you drink more than usual. Weight-loss surgery shrinks the stomach, whether you've had gastric bypass or LAP-BAND® surgery. Our bodies process alcohol differently now and there are some risk factors everyone should be aware of beyond possible addiction.

First of all, alcohol contains a high number of calories and it breaks down vitamins. Alcohol reduces the absorption of vitamins B1, B2, and other B complex vitamins. If you've had gastric bypass surgery, you run greater risks since your body already has difficulty absorbing enough of those vitamins. We don't need an added factor nudging us toward vitamin deficiencies and possible major health issues.

Another problem for gastric bypass patients is that alcohol passes directly from your stomach pouch into your upper gut or jejunum. This second part of the gut has a large surface area, so it absorbs the alcohol rapidly — especially if you've been eating less.

Studies have shown that gastric bypass patients have a significantly higher rate of alcohol absorption than normal. Their blood alcohol reaches higher levels more rapidly and on less alcohol, and the effects last longer. So you can drink one glass of wine and be too impaired to drive a car and have a blood alcohol level high enough to be tagged as a drunk driver. So use great caution if you decide to drink.

When people engage in any addictive behavior, it's because they want and/or need to alter their mood. Two points are important here. The first point is that people who engage in addictive behavior are probably not replacing their addiction to food, just adding another addiction, because their addiction to food is probably lurking within them indefinitely. The second point is that the new addiction is not a result of the gastric surgery; it happens because they have not resolved the issues that led them to develop their addiction to food.

Until they resolve those issues, they will be vulnerable to addiction transfer. And you've got to take steps to avoid joining that crowd.

While you're working on your body, I advise you to work on your head and your heart. Take a look at what issues are behind your eating addiction. Work to resolve those issues, whatever they are.

You can develop healthy, positive addictions. My friends have accused me of becoming addicted to exercise. If it's true, then I'd take that addiction over any other. You can become passionate about a hobby or about social or political causes. There are so many healthy activities to which we can commit our energy. I suggest thinking about the possibilities and finding some that will work for you.

It should be noted that research has revealed that dopamine — a brain chemical associated with addiction to alcohol, cocaine, and other drugs — may also be an important factor in obesity. Dopamine is a neurotransmitter that is involved in producing feelings of satisfaction and pleasure.

Scientists at Brookhaven National Laboratory have determined that obese people have fewer receptors for dopamine. It is yet unknown whether this deficiency is genetic or a result of overeating. But, whatever the cause, it seems that obese people may eat more to try to stimulate their dopamine receptors and increase their pleasure.

The researchers noted that exercise may enable stimulation of the dopamine circuits by increasing the release of dopamine and increasing the number of dopamine receptors. If the results from studies of animals are valid for humans, obese people could boost their dopamine response by exercising. Another good reason to be physically active!

👍*FNM*

10/25/05: My New Life, day 581

I have one more surgery scheduled for December 15. I'll have a breast reduction and lift, which I hope will help with my shoulder, neck, and back pain. I've never been less than a D since the age of 12 and I look forward to carrying less weight up top. I will also have excess skin removed from the inner thighs. Again, I don't look forward to the surgery and recovery, but am eagerly anticipating the results.

Commentary

In the previous chapter I talked about plastic surgery. Breast reductions are often covered by insurance companies because excess weight on top can lead to major back, neck, and shoulder problems. I chose to have my legs done both for aesthetic reasons and because the excess skin got in the way of all my walking and biking. This surgery was not covered and it meant making some financial sacrifices. I felt guilty at first, worried that I was being too vain. But that was the old me talking, a voice in my head from the past. I had worked hard and decided it was OK to take care of myself.

And what if you want to have plastic surgery only for psychological reasons? If you decide to do so, I would advise that you be realistic in your expectations. Just as you should not have expected weight-loss surgery to make your body the perfect shape, you should not expect plastic surgery to give your body a perfect appearance.

👍*FNM*

10/30/05: My New Life, day 586

In our support group last month we talked about mindful eating. At first I thought our facilitator was talking about what I'd learned in my mindful meditation class – to eat slowly, paying attention to each bite – taking in the flavor, texture, and how it nurtures you and makes you feel. That's a good way to eat – when you remember to do it, which I rarely do.

But she was talking about something else. She meant thinking before you eat – before anything goes into your mouth – always being aware of what, why, and when you're eating. Nothing goes into your mouth without thinking about it and making a conscious decision to eat that bite of food. That's the operative word – *conscious*. How much of our eating in the past has been unconscious? Grab a bag of chips and just keep shoveling them in as you watch TV or read a book. How often have you gotten to the end of a meal or snack, looked down at your plate, and thought, "It's gone already," or "I think that tasted pretty good, I'll have to have some more and see," or even "What did I just eat?"

So I've been practicing this kind of mindful eating. I had to keep reminding myself to do this — and I often forgot at first. But it takes practice. Each time I start to go for food or think I need food, I stop and ask myself several questions — Am I hungry? Why do I feel a need to eat right now? Or what am I feeling emotionally? If I am hungry, what am I hungry for? Is that a good choice or are there other choices? I've added another dimension to it: if I realize my hunger is head hunger and I don't really need food, but I decide I really want to have something anyway, I tell myself to wait five or 10 minutes. Every now and then, if I wait, the need to eat will pass.

I'm getting better at remembering and implementing this tool and it's been very helpful. In fact it's almost getting automatic. Part of this process is accepting the fact that sometimes we're going to eat for no good reason but we want to eat. When we're conscious of it, we can have that snack and hopefully move on and not get caught in the cycle of recrimination.

I feel confident that I've made many of the life changes necessary to continue to keep the weight off. Nothing is foolproof, though, and at the suggestion of my good friend, I have support systems in place and a plan set in my mind for those really difficult times when I'm not so confident and things seem to be falling apart. Those times will come. But right now, I feel on top of the world and I'm looking forward to the rest of my life.

Commentary

There are so many little tools that you can find and develop along the way. The Rules of the Pouch give us tools. I've made many suggestions throughout this book. Other books and Web sites will give you ideas. Your support group members are always willing to share what works for them. Try all of these tools and find out what's going to work for you. And what works today might not work tomorrow. Keep searching for ideas and possible answers. Never become complacent and never give up.

👍*FNM*

12/12/05: My New Life, day 629

I've continued to see a psychotherapist. I've been extremely lucky to find a woman who has gone through gastric bypass surgery herself and understands most of the issues I face. I consider this one of my invaluable tools and an important backup for the times life seem to overwhelm me and I want so much to slip back into using food for comfort. She's helping me heal the child/teenager/woman within who felt the need to mask the pain and hurt with food. She also helps me stay focused on what I'm doing that is supporting my new lifestyle and the changes I want to continue to make.

Commentary

If you've allowed your weight to become the biggest issue in your life, the key limitation, the major factor defining your self-image, it's time to change.

Maybe for years you've blamed your weight when you've felt unhappy, depressed, lonely, unable to make many friends, forced to smile and be nice in order to get people to want you around, and all those other tough times.

Well, stop! You're now getting rid of that excuse, that villain. Now you can be free from the problems caused by your weight.

But that means that you will have to deal with other reasons if you still at times feel sad, depressed, lonely, and otherwise bad. If you do not, then you will be making it even more difficult to lose weight and to get into better shape and maintain your better life.

👍*FNM*

Wrap-Up

Once again we need to look at what weight-loss surgery has done for us and what it has not done. If you've had LAP-BAND® surgery, it's restricted your stomach capacity so you eat less. If you've had gastric surgery, it's changed part of your digestive system so your stomach has a much smaller capacity and you absorb fewer of the calories in the food you eat. Weight-loss surgery has helped us to lose a lot of weight in a relatively short time. In other words, it has given us a big jump-start to being thinner and healthier. It has made it easier for us to lose weight and easier to make the changes necessary for long-term success.

What it has not done is change our brains or minds. It's up to us to change our approach to food and exercise — to change the way we live our lives. If we don't make those kinds of changes, we are cutting down drastically on our chances for long-term success in keeping the weight off.

Do you know why you overeat? Do you recognize what emotions, events, or circumstances are triggers for head hunger or emotional eating? Do you eat when you're sad, angry, stressed, lonely, or bored? Do you eat more when it's a family get-together, dinner out, a party, or friends gathering to watch a sporting event? Do you eat mindlessly when reading, sitting at the computer, driving, or at work? Do you find yourself eating more around certain people? These are questions you might want to ask yourself — and then look carefully at your answers.

What can you change? Being aware of the answers is a good first step, but following through with some changes is even better. If you always eat when you crawl into bed to read at night, what could you do differently? You could ask people in your support group what they do, to get some ideas. But often, if you take a little time to think, you have within yourself the answer that will work for you.

Try this:

1. Think of one trigger that causes you to eat.
2. Think of three possible things you could do differently the next time this trigger activates.
3. Choose at least one of those as an action step you can take next time that trigger activates.
4. Tell your action step to someone you trust, someone willing to support your efforts.
5. When you take that action step, report back to that person how it worked or did not work.

If these steps help you modify your behavior, apply them to another trigger.

Finally, I also recommend, as I mentioned in Chapter 2, two books by Geneen Roth that address the emotional issues around eating — *Breaking Free from Emotional Eating* and *When Food Is Love: Exploring the Relationship Between Eating and Intimacy*.

Psychotherapy

As I've mentioned, psychotherapy has been a valuable tool for me. It's a good idea to sit down with your therapist at the beginning and go over what you see as your problem areas, what you want to accomplish, your goals. This can give you a starting point. Your therapist can help you look at some of the issues around why you eat. He or she can help you take a look at ways to deal with the emotional issues around eating and possibly help you change some of your thinking. Your therapist can be an outside sounding board to what might be bringing stress and anxiety into your life.

Self-Talk

We all know about self-talk. We all have those little voices going on inside our heads. Those voices are often tapes from our past. If you listen carefully to what you find yourself saying in your head, especially during times of stress or when we're feeling down or vulnerable, you'll hear the words of your mother, father, grandparent, teacher, boss, or anyone who has been critical, negative, or mentally abusive in your life.

I've heard these voices called many things, but two of my favorites are "monkey mind" and "gremlins." Can't you just imagine those little voices chattering away like monkeys or gremlins?

What you want to do is replace those gremlin voices or negative self-talk with positive self-talk. Give yourself positive feedback, encouragement, pep talks, love, and understanding. Talk your way through difficult situations, down times, moments of weakness, or feelings of inadequacy. And any times you start to hear those little negative voices take over, talk back — tell those other voices where they can go!

Wouldn't it be great to have your own personal cheerleader constantly by your side telling you what a great job you're doing, pointing out all the right things you're doing, encouraging you to get back up when you fall, letting you know how wonderful you are? We can have that personal cheerleader right inside our heads – just let her or him loose and give that cheerleader full rein.

Again, one of the more helpful and fun books I've found on this subject is *Taming Your Gremlin*, by Rick Carson. The subtitle describes what the book offers: "A Surprisingly Simple Method for Getting out of Your Own Way." In a humorous way — "Your gremlin is the sleazy master of misery lurking in the shadows of your very own mind" — this book helps us effectively confront the very serious damage caused by our inner voices.

Affirmations and Visualization

Many of you are familiar with the practice of affirmations. These are positive statements of how you want your life to look. Again, as evidenced in much of the self-help literature today, we attract what we think. If we think, *I am fat and ugly and can't control my eating*, we attract that negative energy into our lives. Whereas, if we think, *I am thin, healthy, and beautiful and I choose foods that support that*, we attract that positive energy. The more you constantly see yourself as thin and see yourself choosing healthy food, the more you become that person. My favorite affirmation that I tell myself constantly is *I am thin and I think and live like a thin person*. I tell myself this numerous times a day.

Some people find it helpful to write out their affirmations. You can make a list — start with at least 10. You don't have to limit it to just affirmations about being thin and losing or maintaining weight. These affirmations can be about any area in your life in which you feel you need to create more positive energy.

Here are some examples to get you started:

• I choose to make healthy choices for my new life.
• I choose to exercise regularly.
• I am confident that I will be fat no more.

Proclaim your affirmations with passion. The more passionate you are about your affirmations, the more effective they can be.

At one point I wrote my affirmations out on brightly colored cards that I taped up around my apartment. Whenever I opened a cupboard or drawer, walked into a room, or looked up from my computer, there was one of my affirmations staring me in the face. After a while, when they started to just blend in with the environment and I wasn't noticing them as much, I took them down and used a different approach.

At that point I'd started receiving coaching and had various conversations and exercises that helped me acknowledge my strengths and all that I was continuing to do toward my goal of being fat no more. One of the exercises was to write down at the end of each day a list of five successes I'd had that day and to acknowledge myself for those successes. This has now become a more active and more practical strategy for me than the affirmations.

One of the things I've found is that there is no one magic action or exercise that has changed the way I think about myself or that helps me stay positive or keeps me successful. Rather, it's a succession of things I've discovered and steps I've taken. I try to be always looking, seeking, working at staying one step ahead when possible — or handling a crisis as it develops.

During those periods when affirmations just were not working for me for various reasons, I found other ways to create the positive thinking and energy I wanted. Some people create affirmation boxes or collages: they fill a box or design a collage of pictures they've cut out from magazines, printed off the Internet, or found in various places, pictures that depict what they want their life to look like.

I'm very visually oriented. Don't tell me how to get somewhere. Show me a map, give me a visual picture of where I'm going and landmarks, and I know I can get there. This applies in so many areas of my life, so visualization is a helpful tool for me. I try to spend a little time on this each day. This can be a quiet time when I can close my eyes and concentrate or, if it's a super busy day, I might have to settle for doing this while I'm doing something else, like taking a bike ride or fixing dinner.

There are so many ways of doing visualizations. Just decide what you want in your life. Then use your imagination to create what you want.

How can you create more positive energy in your life? What fun and creative ways can you come up with to help yourself see the incredible person you are, you're becoming, and you can be?

Life Coaches

Another avenue for making changes in your life is a life coach. Life coaching is a relatively new support system set up to help people succeed in their lives. A life coach is a professional who provides one-on-one support for a person who is trying to make major changes in his or her life.

There are many types of life coaches out there. Businesses have been using coaches for some time to help their employees become more successful. Personal life coaches help people succeed at making progress in their lives.

You want to find a coach who works in the area of health and wellness or whose focus is on lifestyle changes. A coach doesn't look so much at why we do what we do, but rather at helping us find what we can do that will work for us. A coach will sometimes act as a cheerleader, helping you acknowledge all that you're doing right, looking at your successes and helping you discover how to continue succeeding in the areas of your life in which you want to make changes. A coach can help you find what you want to change and how to change it. A good coach helps you find the answers inside yourself and ways to apply those answers.

How do you find a life coach?

The International Coach Federation — a nonprofit organization formed by professionals worldwide who practice business and personal coaching — offers an online directory of coaches (*www.coachfederation. org/ICF*). You can also find a life coach through the Web site of the International Association of Coaching (*www.certifiedcoach.org*).

As guidance in finding a life coach, the International Coach Federation recommends the following:

1. Find out about coaching by reading some of the hundreds of articles written about it in the last few years.
2. Know your objectives for working with a coach.
3. Interview three coaches before making your decision. Ask about their experience, qualifications, and skills. Ask for at least two references.
4. Think in terms of the relationship: you want a connection between you and the coach that feels right.

There are also specialized coaching approaches attached to a person, organization, or book. For example, Rhonda Britten, through her book, *Fearless Living*, has spawned an entire approach to coaching that I personally have found to be very effective (*www.fearlessliving.org*). I highly recommend Co-active Coaching which emphasizes finding the answers within (*www.co-activenetwork.com*). You will run across many different approaches. The secret is not always in the method, but in how it's applied. Personal recommendations are always a plus.

Life coaches usually work over the phone, but they can also work in person or by e-mail. There's no official regulatory standard for life coaching; anyone can claim to be a life coach. There are many coaching training programs and many types of "certification" and "credentials" for coaches. So, when checking the qualifications of any coach you're considering, find out about the sources of any certificates and other credentials and what was required to earn them. Above all, interview any prospects and focus on the potential for a comfortable and beneficial relationship.

I have been on both the giving end and the receiving end of coaching. Through receiving coaching, I've learned a lot about myself and my actions. It's helped me to feel more confident and continue to make changes in my life. Through acting as a life coach, I've become stronger. As I work with other people and their challenges, it thrills me to help them recognize the huge accomplishments they've achieved and how their lives have changed. It also allows me to appreciate my own accomplishments and continually assess what I'm doing that's working or not working. In these ways, coaching has become one of the invaluable tools I'm using to be fat no more.

FNM

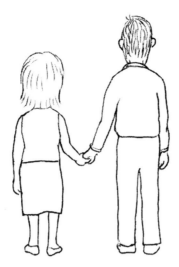

Chapter 15. Relationships

Our family and friends are very important in our efforts to be fat no more. This chapter focuses on our relationships with those around us, our environment — family members and friends, of course, but also the people with whom we work and others in our lives. Every one of your relationships is likely to change, some substantially. For many people who undergo weight-loss surgery, the relationship affected most is with their spouses or partners.

This chapter consists of the stories of nine people who have undergone bariatric surgery. (My story is included among them.) They talk about important relationships in their lives and the effects of their surgery and the resulting changes. The names have been changed.

Story 1: Nicole

I was tall, thin, blonde, and beautiful when I got married. I was also smart and talented. My husband-to-be seemed unintimidated by my smart, professional side. I didn't realize at the time it was because he saw in me great money-earning potential. He wasn't really interested in me as a woman and our marriage deteriorated quickly into a nearly platonic relationship.

For all those years I believed my husband, believed I wasn't beautiful enough or sexy enough to be worth more of his time. He didn't want me and I had to justify that by becoming someone undesirable. I layered on the fat until it made sense that he didn't want me. But I was miserable.

I finally decided that if I was going to be alone, I would rather be alone outside my marriage than alone inside my marriage. I knew I needed to make some changes.

First, I had to lose the weight so I could work again. My health had deteriorated to the point where I couldn't work full time. I had tried to lose in the past, but nothing worked. Surgery seemed to be my remaining avenue. When I got approval for the surgery, I took it as a sign from God that this was my chance to really change my life. Here was my tool. I became unrelentingly driven from the moment I knew I was having the surgery.

I decided I would have the surgery, lose the weight, get back to work full time, handle my health issues, finish building my house, file for divorce, and move out. And I did it all – and all within one year. I felt invincible — until one year after the surgery, when I found the lump and was diagnosed with breast cancer.

When the cancer came along, I knew it would be difficult, but I had the strength to get through it. I had gotten rid of the stone from around my neck (my husband) and was free to nurture myself — say yes to what I needed — and not spend so much of my time and energy fighting and arguing in lose-lose situations. I put my newfound energy into dealing with my cancer — and one year later I am a survivor.

I feel that I'm no longer wasting my life away. I'm there for my children, teaching them through my example what it takes to live life and not give up. My older daughter has dealt with her own weight issues through her childhood and early teens. She was anorexic for a while, because she didn't want to look like me. She has watched me lose the weight and is very proud of me. I think she's learning to make better decisions and be kinder to herself by watching me.

Bariatric surgery has taught me that there's nothing to be gained by giving up — you have to give it your all.

Commentary

Here we have a relationship that was bad from the beginning, based on finances rather than love. And it caused Nicole to change from thin and beautiful to fat and, in her word, "undesirable." As a result, she went from being talented and professional to being in poor health and unable to work full time.

She had to rescue herself, from her obesity and health problems and then from her marriage —even if it meant being alone. As she puts it, she was already alone inside her marriage.

But she had relationships to recover and to strengthen with her children, particularly her older daughter, who was developing weight issues because of her mother. Now, after losing weight through bariatric surgery and surviving breast cancer, she can be an example for them, because of her efforts and what she's accomplished.

👍*FNM*

Story 2: Anna

As I was researching weight-loss surgery, I read and heard that going through bariatric surgery and losing all the weight could have a detrimental affect on a marriage. No way was that going to happen to me! I was not going to be a statistic in failed marriages just because I lost weight! However, inside a small voice was whispering that it was a possibility. But I don't give up easily.

I was in a marriage that had been deteriorating for a number of years. Our relationship had moved from husband/wife to something closer to sometimes friends and more often someone to take all your frustrations out on. There was certainly no romance or intimacy left. My husband was mentally abusive and I didn't believe I deserved or could ever have anything better. I had settled for something less than I wanted in a life partner because I had spent a lifetime being overweight and not being able to attract men who viewed me in a romantic manner. I had finally found a man who seemed to appreciate all aspects of me, including my body.

We were a real team to start with — eating buddies, codependent over-eaters. My husband was dealing with depression and many other major health issues. He felt that he couldn't control much in his life, but he could control me, using anger and guilt. He often threatened suicide or bodily harm to himself if he didn't get his way. He knew my weak spots: I would always respond to someone else being harmed. I was unhappy and at times depressed and spent the last five years wanting to leave. But I was held in place by a feeling of helplessness, worthlessness, and guilt.

After the surgery, as I started to lose the weight, I gained confidence in myself. I began to view myself very differently and began to actually love myself. The more confident I became, the more threatened my husband felt.

He preferred me fat. He wanted a larger woman and I knew that from the start — it was one of the things that brought us together. But I wasn't fat by choice and I had always worked to change that. Now that I had finally fulfilled my dreams, I certainly wasn't willing to give up all that I had achieved — the happiness I found in the freedom of being able to move my body, the energy, happiness, and enthusiasm — just so he could have things as they always were.

I began to stand up for myself and not allow him to control me as much. This made him more angry and more controlling, to the point where there was constant tension and fighting. It took a couple of years after losing the weight before I finally acknowledged the truth of what our relationship had became and had the confidence to walk away.

It wasn't easy: it triggered a lot of guilt, loss, and financial and emotional stress. All the good food and exercise habits I had put in place were challenged to the max.

But I'm finding the strength within myself to handle each day as it comes and stand up for what I know is healthy for me. I'm enjoying the freedom to remake my life the way I want it to be and have relationships that support the new strong, loving, healthy me.

Commentary

This seems to be a typical result when the "new" person changes and the partner refuses to adapt and clings to the past, to the history of the relationship.

Anna is intelligent, personable, educated, cultured, enthusiastic, and attractive and she has a good sense of humor. But from early on she was limited by her weight. In high school she was always everybody's friend, because boys could associate with her without making their girlfriends jealous and girls felt comfortable with her because they didn't consider her a threat. She could have had her pick of the boys except for her size. After high school, it was the same story: Anna had lots of friends, but not much romance. As she says, "I had settled for something less than I wanted in a life partner because I had spent a lifetime being overweight and not being able to attract men who viewed me in a romantic manner."

According to another person who chose weight-loss surgery, many married people who undergo WLS may have settled for less than they wanted in a partner, because they needed affection and were tired or afraid of being alone. The partner may have wanted the relationship for reasons that could be considered unhealthy, perhaps out of pity, perhaps because the partner also had weight problems, or perhaps because he or she had psychological or emotional issues, such as a need to dominate or a need for security. (There can be a certain security and feeling of control in being involved with a person who seems to have few options.) The relationship may be unsatisfactory, to one or both of them, but it continues. Then, after WLS and a subsequent transformation, the "new" person leaves the marriage and moves on. (In fact, in some cases, that's one of the person's goals.) When one person in a close relationship changes, his or her partner must adapt or their relationship may end.

For Anna, the relationship had been dying for years and she and her husband were endangering their lives by remaining obese and accepting obesity as their fate. She chose to rescue herself from that fate. Her husband chose not to change.

☝*FNM*

Story 3: Rita

Well, I must say it has been quite a year. I have been married for 21 years. My husband and I have two boys, 19 and 16. Our marriage hasn't been up to par for the last 10 years or so; we have just sort of gone our separate ways. My husband is a bowler and used to schedule tournaments almost every weekend. We haven't taken a vacation together in over 10 years. He goes away for the tourneys all the time without me or the boys.

My world changed on August 28, 2006. I had gastric bypass surgery. It changed my whole world.

I started losing weight immediately and began to feel more confident about myself and noticing my surroundings weren't what they should be. My children always asked me, "Mom, why do you put up with

Dad's crap?" They knew something was wrong. My husband was a sports addict. When he wasn't working, you could find him in his leather recliner eating huge bowls of popcorn and watching some type of sports on TV. He never really noticed when I came or went.

That all changed in February of 2007. I was helping a friend who holds auctions for families that have lost a family member or are moving, etc. I play like Vanna White and hold up the items that are up for bid. I saw a man from across the room and knew that I just had to meet him. That changed my life dramatically from the life I knew.

We met. He was with three other men. We went to dinner that night, all four of us, and had a great time. Then he and I had dinner, lunch, and breakfast together for the next two weeks. I realized that there was more to life than sports and a husband who ignores me. I was actually being given compliments, being treated with respect, taken out to eat, strolls along the lake. It was wonderful.

I came home one night and told my husband that I was through with our marriage and that I wanted to move out. He didn't seem to care one way or another. I moved out on February 21, 2007.

I felt so independent, paying my own bills, being responsible for myself, breaking away from the unhappiness I have felt for years and living life like I felt I should be living it.

The boyfriend and I got closer. He eventually moved in with me. He had a lot of baggage associated with him. It was getting harder to get along with him. Finally in May we broke it off, although we still had strong feelings for each other. We saw each other occasionally, but just as friends. I joined a few online singles clubs. I had a few dates, but they all wanted to get too serious. I just wanted someone to go places with, to spend time with — nothing serious.

During all of this time, my husband started reading relationship books — eight, to be exact. He also talked with his doctor about a therapist. His doctor recommended one from a church in town. He started seeing her and that's when he began to change. He also started journaling daily.

Since February we talked several times a week, but I didn't want to hear how much he loved me or wanted me back. I just wanted to be left alone, live my life by myself.

He never gave up. He continued to read whatever he could get his hands on, talk to whoever he could about our situation and what he could do to make things right.

Around July he started calling more and we began doing things together as friends. I made that very clear. I noticed a huge change in him. He lost 50 lbs. He treated me with respect. He listened when I talked. He wanted to go places with me, to experience what I was experiencing. It was all so new to me. He was never like this before.

Towards the end of July, I noticed I started having feelings for my husband again, feelings that had been gone for years. I found him attractive again. I found myself wanting him in ways I have not wanted him before. We started dating and by the end of August I moved back home. Yes, home!

It feels so good to be back home with my family. In a home where there is abundant love and respect for each other. My husband and I do almost everything together. He quit eating popcorn constantly, quit watching so much sports on TV. We lie in bed and read quietly, just as long as we are together. He finds me very attractive.

I have this new confidence about myself. I hold my head up high now. I no longer feel I am hiding behind nearly 200 lbs. of excess weight that has disappeared forever. I am so thankful for RNY surgery. It has changed my life forever.

Commentary

This story is similar to the story told by Anna, except that Rita's husband chose to adapt. At first, "he didn't seem to care one way or another." But then he started reading about relationships, working with a therapist, and journaling. It was truly a self-improvement project. And he persisted in pursuing Rita, even though she resisted, insisting that she wanted to live without him. "He never gave up" in his quest to do "what he could do to make things right."

And it worked out for him and for Rita. After her surgery, she decided that she deserved the chance to find something better for herself, a better relationship. She enjoyed her independence — and then she found something better, a better relationship, because her husband decided that he loved her enough to improve and to work on forming a new relationship.

Story 4: Claudette

I never had a weight problem until I started having kids. I have two children — 5 and 8. I never lost the "baby weight" after each pregnancy. This became a very sticky point between my husband and me. He had no clue what I went through physically, emotionally, and hormonally during and after the pregnancies. It wasn't like I didn't try to lose the weight!

I went through months and months of almost no sleep, with the added stress of going back to a full-time job after two months each time, doing the larger portion of the housekeeping and all the cooking, dropping the kids off and picking them up from day care, and often doing all this for a week at a time when my husband was traveling for business.

Our sex life dribbled off into nothing. We never had time alone anymore and when we did we usually ended up fighting about my weight. I must admit, I didn't do much to enhance my looks during that time — I didn't have the energy and I was disgusted by how I looked, mostly wearing tent-like clothes that hid the fat.

My sister had weight-loss surgery and was looking fabulous. She helped talk me through the fear and helped me make the decision to go ahead. My husband was all for it.

It was the best decision I ever made. I lost 140 pounds and was back down to my pre-pregnancy weight and feeling really good about myself. My husband was thrilled to have his old wife back.

I found that I had a confidence in myself that I hadn't had since I was in my early 20s. I also found that men were responding to me in a way they hadn't since I was in my 20s either. It was flattering and irresistible. I couldn't help but respond to all the attention I was getting and would invariably flirt back. My husband started to get jealous. I never took any of the flirtations past a certain point, but he was afraid I would.

We started getting counseling to deal with these issues. I've also gotten individual counseling to deal with all the issues that have come up around my eating. We're working on it — and most of the time I'm confident we're going to make it. But I have to admit that there are days when I'd like to take that flirting past the safe stage.

I don't know for sure what the future holds right now. All I know is that I'm enjoying feeling like a woman again and I don't want to lose that.

Commentary

It can be such a temptation to benefit more fully from looking and feeling good again after years of being overweight. As Claudette says of the attention she attracted from men, "It was flattering and irresistible. I couldn't help but respond to all the attention I was getting and would invariably flirt back."

Sometimes reactions to the attention become extreme. Some people after weight-loss surgery develop a transfer addiction to sex. This is particularly likely if they have not been receiving attention from their spouse or significant other or from anybody at all, such as was the case with Claudette. Another woman, in confessing some concern about a transfer addiction as she was returning to her younger weight, "I think my addiction may have become sex or maybe it's been so long since I have been given attention that it is a coincidence. I don't know, but I'm totally loving it."

Claudette had the support of her husband in her decision to undergo surgery and he was pleased with the results, "thrilled to have his old wife back." Even though her weight gain has started only eight years earlier and had become "a very sticky point" in that time, they were not prepared for all the effects of her success in losing weight. They did not anticipate how she would feel, how deprived of attention she had felt during those eight years. She had lost so much, but gradually, so she may not have realized how she would react to returning to her earlier body.

👍*FNM*

Story 5: Deborah

I shattered my ankle in October 1996 and have walked in pain since. Being overweight didn't help. About five years ago, I blew out my other foot compensating for the ankle, then developed bone spurs in my heels. It was to the point I would crawl. I saw a man in the grocery store walking on pegs and decided I could do that. He looked to be pain-free. That's when I went to a podiatrist. He didn't help. So I continued to suffer.

In the meantime, several people that I know have had the bypass surgery successfully. I talked to my husband about it. After the surgery seminar, we decided that if it could help me walk it would be worth it. And the side effects were a lot nicer than cutting off my legs. I not only talked to friends and family beforehand, but also my customers. I discovered many of them already had it. I have always had a huge support team with friends and family and customers. My mother worried I would starve to death, but has since changed her opinion of the surgery.

As for affecting my personal relationships, nothing has changed except that I am able to walk circles around my dad for the first time in many years.

It will be one year since the surgery on January 4 and the reactions of friends, family, and customers have been very positive. My main concern is losing too much. I have lost 109 lbs. and have about six more months of weight loss ahead of me. I don't need to lose any more. I have noticed that pattern in friends who have had the surgery but then tend to level off.

People are still surprised at my weight loss and compliment the new me. I have been fortunate to have such a life and so many supportive people in it. The fact that my relationships have remained the same only proves to me how solid they are and the people in my life are there because they want to be.

Commentary

This is a wonderful success story. In her decision to undergo surgery, Deborah received support from her husband and from friends, family, and even customers of her store. Of course, if the alternative is pain and immobility, weight-loss surgery is likely to generate a more positive reaction and more support than if the effects of obesity are less obvious. And someone who can hardly walk is less likely to be accused of "taking the easy way out" rather than losing weight "the old-fashioned way."

Deborah makes an excellent point: "I have been fortunate to have ... so many supportive people .... The fact that my relationships have remained the same only proves to me how solid they are and the people in my life are there because they want to be."

Story 6: Terri and Lynda

When I first told my partner, Lynda, I was thinking about bariatric surgery, she was angry.

It wasn't the reaction I expected. We had been together for five years and both struggled with our weight. I was 29 years old, had just been diagnosed with high blood pressure, and weighed over 400 pounds.

As the weeks went by, I knew I had to make a decision about surgery with or without Lynda's support. Lynda was my best friend and the love of my life, but we also supported each other's overeating and lack of self-care. Even though we're both educated professionals, we were destroying our bodies with the excess weight, and something had to give. Deep down, I knew Lynda wasn't angry, she was afraid — afraid of the fact I'd have to undergo surgery and afraid that I would leave her behind on a journey to health. However, I knew that once I began the surgery process she would hang back and check it out and then have it herself.

I was approved for LAP-BAND® surgery on February 2, 2006. Lynda listened to me while I was on the phone with my doctor's office, picking a date for my surgery. After I hung up, she told me that she had been doing a lot of thinking and that she wanted to have the band as well.

I had my procedure March 16, 2006 and Lynda had her procedure done July 7, 2006. The entire bariatric process is more psychological than anything. My problem was that I ate way too much, I was addicted to food, and only true commitment could change that. But I also knew that the dynamic between Lynda and me would have to change, too. We ate when we were upset, we ate when we were happy, we ate when we were bored. We both watched each other struggle to breathe as we climbed a flight of stairs, but we also called each other on the phone during a drive home from work to ask what the fast food craving for the evening was. It's bad enough to deal with an addiction on your own, but when there is someone else to fuel it, I really believe that they both have to change or go their separate ways.

While Lynda and I were able to support each other and, best of all, be able to relate to the physical and psychological challenges and experiences unique to bariatric surgery, we had to realize that we had to stick to what worked best for us. Everyone's bariatric journey is slightly different.

It was hard for us to truly understand that at first. I was jealous because Lynda could eat a number of foods that I couldn't. (Some foods just can't go through my band.) Lynda had a really hard time losing the weight, even though she ate well and exercised. Because I am much bigger than Lynda, about a foot taller and 150 pounds heavier, I lost weight much faster than she did and she was jealous. It never became a competition; we would just beat ourselves up when we compared our successes and we each felt our own wasn't as good. We talked about it a lot and had to agree that we're two different people with two very different bodies; we even had different exercise needs and had to work out separately.

I was very happy to have someone to ride the wave with. We expected our relationship with each other to change. But we were very surprised at how much our surgeries impacted our parents and close family. Many of them gave us endless sympathy. Lynda and I couldn't figure out why our families felt sorry for us — and constantly told us so — because we had to eat so little and had to miss out on carbonated beverages. Lynda's aunt told us she could never have the surgery because she would "die" without Diet Coke. Lynda was very close to her grandmother, but both of our feelings were hurt when her grandmother insisted that we shouldn't have had the surgery and we could have done it if we just ate right and exercised.

Even though both of our families consist of mainly overweight people, no one understood the psychological land mine of food addiction. I was very lucky to have a partner who not only understood it, but was also willing to make conquering that land-mine part of our relationship.

Half of our families pitied us and the other half thought the surgery was a cop-out. It made us very self-conscious. It took a long time for them not to pay attention to how little we ate. We also discovered our change made other people uncomfortable and, in the long run, you cannot and should not feel guilty about this journey. You have to take care of yourself first. Everything else is secondary.

After 18 months, Lynda lost almost 100 pounds, with about 40 more to go. As for me, I lost 120 pounds in the first 11 months after surgery, but put my weight-loss journey on hold to become pregnant. Our daughter was born October 24, 2007. I still have about 80 more pounds to go.

Commentary

This is a beautiful success story. Terri and Lynda are making it work out happily because they communicate well and they're both committed.

But this story started because Terri was determined to change her life "with or without Lynda's support," determined to break free from their shared problem with "overeating and lack of self-care." She recognized that the dynamic between them had to change:

"It's bad enough to deal with an addiction on your own, but when there is someone else to fuel it, I really believe that they both have to change or go their separate ways."

Terri and Lynda discussed working on the problem together, but they were smart and strong enough to agree that they had to work on it in different ways. It can be harder for partners to work on a common weight problem together in spirit but separately in body.

They expected their relationship would change and they prepared for those changes. However, they were not prepared for the reactions of their families, for the mix of pity and disapproval from "mainly overweight people" who, ironically, did not understand "the psychological land mine of food addiction." They were also not prepared for the discomfort they would be causing others. However, Terri's words could serve as a mantra for anybody considering weight-loss surgery: "You have to take care of yourself first. Everything else is secondary."

Terri and Lynda went through surgery together and they've been making the weight-loss journey together, on separate but parallel paths. And now they are raising a daughter – and even though her parents both come from families of "mainly overweight people," you can bet that their daughter will not be allowed to become a victim of the addiction to eating.

👍*FNM*

Story 7: Mary Ann

I battled with my weight through most of my teens, but managed to keep it somewhat under control. When I met my husband at age 23, I wasn't exactly skinny, but I wasn't fat either. He always said I was just right.

It was love at first sight and we were married a year later. We both loved kids, wanted a big family, and had our first child right away. We were thrilled and couldn't wait to have more.

I put on a quite a bit of weight through my pregnancy and couldn't get it off afterwards. In fact, the weight kept piling on. I was a busy full-time mommy — home all day — and the fridge and cupboards were too convenient. In the meantime, we were trying to have a second child, with no luck.

My husband was so supportive and understanding and never gave me a hard time about my weight, but I could see that it was putting stress on our relationship because I was unhappy. We both understood that the added weight was why I wasn't able to get pregnant again and I had also been diagnosed with diabetes.

I continued to gain weight and it became difficult to get down on the floor and play with my little girl and run around after her. I could see all that I had dreamed of — all that brought joy into my life — slipping away. Yet I couldn't get a handle on my weight. I tried following every program out there, but nothing worked.

Finally, after five years of misery and reaching 360 pounds, I brought up weight-loss surgery to my husband. We read everything we could on the subject, spending a lot of time going over complication and mortality statistics. My husband couldn't bear the thought of losing me and I couldn't bear the thought of leaving my little girl behind. We talked to the surgeons at the local program and were reassured. I wanted to do this and, even though my husband was concerned, he loved me enough to stand behind my decision.

The surgery was a huge success and I lost 220 pounds in one year! No more diabetes, I had boundless energy and spent my days running around with my little girl, and my husband and I were like young lovers again.

All my friends and family were so happy for me. Happiest of all was my father. My mother had passed when I was in my early teens and my father and I became a team. We meant the world to each other. I guess I inherited my weight problems from my dad. I was hoping that my weight loss might spur him on to consider the surgery. He had numerous health problems due to his weight and I told him I didn't want to lose him too. One year after my surgery, my dad decided to follow in my footsteps and go through bariatric surgery.

I had been cautioned not to get pregnant for two years following the surgery, but I was doing so well and after 16 months it just happened. We were thrilled and just over two years after my surgery we had a second daughter. One of the happiest days of my life was the day our second daughter was christened. I stood between my loving husband and my beaming thin and fit father with my new baby in my arms and my older daughter running circles around us. It was like a fairy tale. I know life isn't always perfect — but this felt as close as it can get.

Commentary

This is as good as it gets, "like a fairy tale," as Mary Ann puts it.

Mary Ann was lucky in many ways, yes, but she did some smart things to make the most of her luck in terms of her relationships. She was fortunate to have a good, solid, loving relationship with her husband, but she also was wise to involve him in her weight-loss experience from the start, getting his support for the difficult journey. She was fortunate to have a father who supported her efforts and was open to learning from his daughter's example, but she was wise not to push him into bariatric surgery.

Whatever we have through fortune, we can lose if we're not smart. And if we're smart, we can make the most of our fortune. We can choose not to blame our genes, our environment, and the people in our lives. We can make the decision to be fat no more.

FNM

Conclusions About Relationships

As mentioned earlier and as some of these stories show, relationships with spouses or partners can change substantially. You may find that your surgery and weight loss result in one or more of the following changes in your relationship:

• My partner fails to notice and appreciate that I am losing weight, becoming more active physically, eating healthier, and generally improving.

• My partner worries about losing the security of feeling that I'm "safe," that is, less attractive.

• My partner is afraid of not being able to keep up with me.

- My partner is treating me better, with more respect and love.
- My partner undermines my efforts to lose weight, intentionally or unintentionally.
- My partner seems to be feeling less self-confident as I gain confidence in myself.
- My partner finds my loose skin unattractive.
- My partner wants to be sexually more active.
- My partner wants to be sexually less active.
- My partner is suggesting that I get some plastic surgery.
- My partner is opposed to my getting any plastic surgery.
- My partner objects to my new eating behaviors at home.
- My partner is becoming more concerned about his/her physical condition and health.
- My partner is frustrated that I am avoiding social situations centered on eating and drinking.
- My partner is annoyed that we now keep few or no junk foods around the house.
- My partner is proud of the self-discipline I'm showing in eating healthier and getting into better shape.
- My partner is enthusiastic about joining me in walking and other physical activities.
- My partner resents the fact that members of my support group are so important in my life.
- My partner complains that some of our friends are less available since I started changing my life.
- My partner claims that I'm not as nice as when I was heavier.
- My partner seems jealous that I'm getting into better shape and enjoying life more.
- My partner is paying more attention to foods when shopping and making healthier food choices our family.

Friendships and Work Relationships

Friendships and work relationships can also be affected as you change your life. The dynamics will start changing as soon as you undergo weight-loss surgery and begin losing weight and becoming more fit.

Some or most or even all of your friends may think that you're happier, more active, and more enthusiastic. But there may be others who think that it's less enjoyable to be around you, especially if the activities you've enjoyed together have involved eating and drinking.

As you change, some of the other people in your life may feel pressure to change, too — and they may react well or not so well. "Now that you're eating differently, I guess we can't go to the same restaurants for lunch." "Hmm, now I suppose I should try to lose some weight, too."

As you engage in more interests, such as dating or physical activities, and meet other people, some of your old friends will likely have a smaller place in your life. You'll probably have less time to spend with them — and may be less interested in being with them as you develop more options.

At work, you may be more energetic and work harder and more enthusiastically — but you also may have more reasons to leave on time, to not be willing or able to stay late. If you start bringing your lunch, you'll miss out on the socializing that happens when co-workers go out to eat. If you choose to eat in a restaurant, you may be eating alone or with fewer co-workers if the restaurants you choose don't have the foods that the others prefer.

These are just a few of the effects that you can expect from all of the changes you'll be making in your life, changes that will require adjustments, both for you and for the people in your life.

What can you do to minimize the negative effects of the changes you're making in your life?

Think about each of your relationships and how it will probably or possibly be affected.

Prepare your family members, friends, co-workers, and others for your new life — and prepare yourself for their reactions.

Communicate about what you're doing and how you want your life to change — and be honest about the possible effects on your relationships.

Expect that some people who seem positive about your goals and promise to support you in your efforts may become less supportive.

Thank the people in your life for whatever they do to support your efforts to live healthier. Let them know how much you appreciate them. Those who help you deserve thanks — and are more likely to continue to help you.

Work on keeping and improving relationships with the people who matter most to you.

Be especially considerate of your partner, family members, friends, and co-workers. They may be unsure of how you're changing and how the changes will affect them. Paying special attention should reassure them.

Be attentive to any concerns that family members, friends, and co-workers may express about changes in your personality and behavior. Don't be offended or become defensive. You're experiencing the changes from within and you're probably very focused on them. It's good to know how others are reacting to the new you.

Don't talk too much about your surgery or weight loss. Show interest in what the people in your life are doing.

Involve others in your new life, but don't impose it on them. Include your partner, family members, and friends in your new activities — but only if they express interest. Don't expect them to embrace your activities with as much enthusiasm as you may feel. And be open to suggestions of activities from those around you, especially if you've been unable or unwilling to participate in such activities in the past.

Make your partner feel special, with loving attention. As you change in your new life, your partner may feel unsure or insecure about your relationship. Whether this happens or not, it's always good to reassure.

Consider getting couples therapy if your relationship becomes more difficult. Be sensitive if you believe that therapy might help; your partner may not be as interested or open to therapy — and likely less if you seem to be demanding or imposing it.

Meet with members of your support groups, either in regular meetings or individually. These are people who understand what you're experiencing.

Form other relationships — particularly with people who are devoted to being physically fit. A good way to do this is by talking with others in your health club when you exercise or with people whom you meet while walking or biking.

Finally, if you cannot maintain your most important relationships, if you cannot have it all, choose yourself.

Dealing with Feelings

Relationship problems can cause stress and depression, which can cause you to stop losing weight and to start gaining. You may neglect to follow the guidelines for eating healthy and exercising.

If you begin to gain weight because you feel depressed, try to exercise more, focus on the pouch rules, discuss your situation with your support group, and consider getting into counseling.

There's recent evidence that perhaps counseling should be the first resort. An article in the October 2007 issue of *Archives of Surgery* reported that researchers have found "a substantial excess" in deaths from suicide and coronary heart disease among patients who have undergone bariatric surgery.

The researchers checked the records of 16,683 patients in Pennsylvania who had bariatric surgery performed between 1995 and 2004. There were 440 deaths, a mortality rate of 2.6%. Even after the researchers excluded procedure-related deaths that occurred within 30 days after the operation, age- and sex-specific death rates were significantly higher for the study group than for the general Pennsylvania population.

Coronary heart disease was the leading cause of death, accounting for 20% of those deaths. That's probably to be expected. But 16 deaths (4% of the total) were attributable to suicide and another 14 deaths (3% of the total) were overdoses not classified as suicides, which could have been misclassified: "It is very likely that the suicide deaths were ... underestimated because some of the deaths were listed as drug overdoses rather than suicide on the death certificate." In the general population, in a group of this size, only two deaths from suicide would have been expected.

The higher death rates found in the study were likely due to complications caused by obesity itself. In other words, if you're suffering from heart disease, weight-loss surgery will not cure it. If you're suffering from depression, don't expect surgery to deliver you from that darkness.

Earlier in the book, I cautioned against setting your expectations too high. Your excess weight may be your biggest problem, but unless it's your only problem, don't expect that by losing weight you can make your life wonderful. More specifically, don't expect that your relationships will improve or that you'll make lots of new friends.

Preparing for Changes — Anticipated and Unexpected

You can expect that all of your personal relationships after you undergo weight-loss surgery and as you lose weight. The changes in your life will affect all your relationships, but especially your relationship with your spouse or significant other. The percentage of people who get divorced within the first two years after they undergo weight-loss surgery is very high.

Understand that surgery will change more than your body and how you feel about yourself and what you will be able to do. If you are married or in a comparable relationship, think seriously about how the two of you might react to the anticipated changes. If you suspect problems or if you feel unsure, it might be wise to engage in couples counseling to prepare for your surgery. This is true particularly if you have been suffering from low self-esteem, if you feel like you've settled for a less satisfactory relationship because of your weight, if your partner doesn't appreciate you as much as you would like, if your relationship has remained the same for a long time, or if your partner also has a weight problem.

Other close personal relationships can also experience difficult changes. Parents and children of weight-loss surgery patients have often expressed a sense of loss or even regret as their loved ones lose weight and undergo other changes, physical and psychological. Expect your attitude and your interests and your actions and interactions to change — and expect that some people close to you might not be totally positive and supportive as these changes make you a different person from their perspective.

FNM

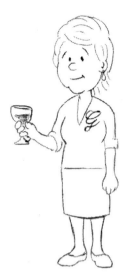

Chapter 16. Enjoy Your New Life, Fat No More

May 2007

Recently I celebrated the three-year anniversary of my new life. On March 23, 2004, weighing 327 pounds, I had bariatric surgery. I had the surgery not just because I was overweight. I had the surgery primarily because I was facing the possibility of major health issues, such as diabetes, back and joint problems, high blood pressure, and heart disease. I detested my body, my inability to move freely and participate in life the way I wanted.

Over the past three years, I've lost 180 pounds, I have no major health issues, I am physically fit, and I celebrate the body I have and what it can do. I have my life back.

However, the work is never done. Having the surgery and losing the weight are only the first step. Then there's the rest of your life!

Is this a success story? I believe so — that's what matters most. Everyone's journey following weight-loss surgery is different and each one measures their own success in different ways.

Was it easy? No, it was hard work and continues to be hard work. I struggle at times and wonder if I can maintain. I battle with my food-addiction demons and sometimes lose. But when I stay focused on the big picture, I know I'm winning.

Has it been worth it? A resounding yes! There are so many things I can do today, seemingly little things like sit in any chair I want, run up a flight of stairs, ride a bicycle, run around the room playing games with my students, not worry about how far I have to walk when going on an outing with friends, etc. I could fill a dozen pages with these types of changes.

But perhaps a more important change is how I feel about myself. I believe in myself, love myself most days, and believe I can do anything I set my mind to. No, these feelings weren't completely absent from my life before, but they were considerably overshadowed by my size. As my body got smaller, my belief in myself got bigger.

There are a few basic principles that I've tried to stay focused on over the past three years and hope to keep in place for the rest of my life.

I believe in myself and forgive myself.

Old habits of getting down on myself when I eat too much, use food for emotional support, skip the exercise for several days, or fail to follow my own basic principles can quickly start me on the old downward spiral of self-loathing, eating, more self-loathing, more eating, etc. When I can forgive myself, believe in myself, let it go, and move on, I can stay out of the dangerous place that is still lurking on the edges of my new lifestyle.

I maintain a strong support network.

My support network includes two bariatric support groups, a psychologist, and positive and supportive friends and family members.

I stay physically active.

For me, this is probably the most important key to maintaining my weight loss.

I continue to emphasize proteins and avoid simple carbohydrates.

When I start eating more carbohydrates, I crave more carbs until all I want are carbs. I still avoid sugar and other simple carbohydrates. It's a rule I set for myself and it's worked so far.

The joys, changes, growth, and consequences of massive weight loss are numerous and extensive. I never imagined how dramatically this would change my life. I don't think there is an area of my life this hasn't touched.

The physical changes I've gone through were only the beginning. There's a popular saying that you have to change from the inside out. But the rapid and dramatic weight loss has pushed me to change from the outside in. As my body changed, I became stronger and more confident. It's an ongoing process as I continue to grow into my new life.

All the changes forced me to re-evaluate so much about my life. This is a good thing, but it's difficult — even painful. Many of my relationships changed, the most significant being my marriage. Any relationship has to be very strong to go through that amount of change. Problems in our marriage that we were willing to accept because we felt we had no other options suddenly pushed us into making decisions. As I was losing weight, I was gaining options. In beginning work on my book, *Fat No More*, I've talked with many other bariatric patients. Similar stories have emerged of people facing major decisions such as ending a relationship. It's one of the possible consequences. I had to face who I was before and who I was becoming and I didn't want to move backward.

Someone asked me once if looking at my "before" pictures bothered me. Sort of — they're a little hard to look at because they make me sad for the little girl/teenager/young woman who was fighting for so long to escape from that large body. But I also look at those pictures and recognize the me that's always been there — the same me that resides in this smaller body now. In many ways I haven't changed — I'm still basically the same person. I can't disown or be ashamed of who I was before — that would make my whole life up to now less than it was. Those pictures also act as a reminder of how far I've come — and how far I could fall if I don't stay vigilant.

Today I feel strong and free in mind, body, and spirit. Free from the prison that was my body. Free to live a fuller life and pursue my dreams.

👍*FNM*

Life is a process and an adventure. Remember to be present in each moment. Enjoy each step in the journey that is your new life. Live, eat, think, and move like the healthy person you are now and you will continue to be that person — fat no more.

Good luck and best wishes!

👍*FNM*

Your Pouch Rules!

(Keys to Long-Term Success Following Roux-en-Y Gastric Bypass)

Jon Gould, M.D., and Michael Garren, M.D.

We have all heard stories about gastric bypass patients who lost a lot of weight after surgery, only to see the pounds creep back on in the years that follow. While a minimal amount of weight regain is common between two and five years after surgery, you should never regain weight to the point at which it once again begins to affect your health and overall quality of life.

The blame for this scenario is frequently assigned to the patient, but all too often poor dietary compliance and a lack of exercise are only part of the story. Unless patients have been properly informed of what they need to do to lose weight, it is unlikely that they will succeed in the long run. Successfully achieving a healthy weight one year after surgery is a nice outcome, but the holy grail of gastric bypass surgery should be a sustained healthy weight after 10, 20, even 30 years!

We bariatric surgeons are fond of saying, "Your pouch is a tool. Learn how it works and use it!" The dictionary defines a tool as "an object used to accomplish a task." Much like a surgical scalpel, your pouch is an ineffective tool unless you know how to properly use it. The following is a summary of what we feel are the keys to achieving the best and longest-lasting results after gastric bypass surgery.

The following rules are intended for those who are more than six to 12 months out from their surgical procedure. Trying to use these rules too soon may be dangerous. Most patients in the first six months after surgery still struggle with achieving their fluid- and protein-intake goals.

Specific goals and strategies for meeting them are outlined in the UW Health Bariatric Surgery Diet Plan. This diet plan is available in printed format or may be downloaded at *www.uwhealth.org/bariatric surgery*. Until you are comfortably achieving these goals each and every day, you should continue to follow the diet as outlined in the diet plan handout and by your dietician. A good time to begin practicing and adhering to the rules of the pouch is when your appetite returns and you are beginning to feel less restricted (easily full).

Things That We Consider in Surgery When We Are Making Your Pouch

Pouch size. A small pouch made from the thick part of your upper stomach (lesser curve) is essential to weight loss. Your new pouch is measured in surgery to be 20-30 mL (one ounce) — about the size of an egg.

Through experience, we have learned that this size pouch is created by dividing the stomach starting on the lesser curve at a point 2-3 cm beyond the junction of the esophagus and the stomach. We use a 25-mm circular stapler to create this connection and therefore the internal diameter of the tubular pouch is 2.5 cm. These dimensions translate into a pouch of roughly 20-30 mL.

The father of bariatric surgery in this country, Dr. Edward Mason, performed a series of experiments on his patients and their pouches. He found that all pouches grew in size during the first two years after surgery. Most pouches ended up with a capacity of about six ounces (180 mL). Some pouches were as big as nine to 10 ounces. Interestingly, the size of each patient's pouch (up to about 12 ounces or 1.5 cups) did not correlate with weight loss. It turns out that for weight maintenance how a pouch is used is more important than how small it is.

Pouch outlet. Your pouch outlet diameter should be small. If we make the connection between your Roux-limb and your pouch (*gastrojejunostomy*) too large, your pouch will empty too quickly after you eat and you will feel hungry again too soon. By using the circular stapler to create our gastrojejunostomy, we create an outlet with an internal diameter of precisely 15 mm every time.

Roux-limb length. The importance of Roux-limb length in weight loss has been widely debated. This is probably much less important for weight loss and maintenance than the size of the pouch or the size of the pouch outlet. Our approach has been to give patients with a BMI less than 50 a 100-cm limb. Everybody else gets a 150-cm Roux limb. Neither length is technically considered a 'long-limb' bypass.

A Simplified Way of Looking at Your Weight (Before and After Bariatric Surgery)

• The goal of every bariatric surgery is to assist in reducing daily caloric intake.

• Surgery levels the playing field, making it possible for you to control your weight.

What Drives You to Eat? ("How Is My Appetite Regulated?")

Appetite regulation is a complex and poorly understood process. Many nervous and hormonal pathways play a role. There are stretch receptors in your stomach pouch that send a signal to your brain that you have eaten enough and your pouch is full. At this point, you should feel satiated. When your pouch empties, your appetite will soon return. When you realize this, you'll know that if you can fill your pouch with low-calorie foods that will empty very slowly, then at the end of the day you will have restricted your caloric intake to a point where you use the equations above to your advantage.

Observations from Successful Patients and Bariatric Surgeons

• Getting a sense of fullness with each meal is essential to success. Avoid grazing.

• Regular meals larger than 12 ounces will eventually result in weight gain.

• Lightly stretching the pouch sends a signal to your brain that you do not need any more food.

• Maintaining that sense of fullness requires keeping the pouch stretched for a while.

• Fasting for more than eight hours will lead to a profound sense of hunger.

• "Soft foods" empty from the pouch quickly. "Heavy" foods empty more slowly.

- Meat and slightly cooked or raw vegetables are good for you and empty very slowly from the pouch.

- Patients who exercise regularly lose more weight and maintain that weight loss longer.

- Bariatric surgery programs that provide long-term support and follow-up and patients who participate in follow-up care and support groups have the best and most durable results.

Your Pouch Rules(!)

1. Meals must be timed about five hours apart or you will become too hungry.

2. You should eat your entire meal in 10-15 minutes. This is contrary to what we told you immediately after your operation. While your pouch was healing, we emphasized tiny bites, thorough chewing, and long meal times (30-45 minutes). Now that your pouch is mature and your appetite has returned, eating quickly will help you to restrict your intake effectively. Eating small bites very slowly allows your pouch to slowly empty out one side as you fill the other. The end result is much larger meal and calorie consumption.

3. No liquids for one and a half to two hours after each meal. This is the same principle as above. Fluids wash your meal out of your pouch. Delaying fluid consumption for this amount of time after filling your pouch allows your pouch to remain full for a long period of time. This prevents your appetite from returning prematurely.

4. After two hours, begin slowly sipping fluids and gradually increase the rate of fluid intake until shortly before your next meal. Your fluid requirements are the same as they have always been. You still need a minimum of 64 ounces (eight cups) of fluid a day (more depending on factors such as exercise, activity, and temperature). This fluid goal requires a special strategy to achieve and still comply with rule #3.

5. Water loading can help you buy time and ward off your appetite between meals. Drinking as much water as fast as

possible will produce a strong sense of fullness. This should last for about 20 minutes.

With practice, the above rules and practices should become second nature.

Avoid absolutes. Special occasions or momentary weaknesses happen to us all. Don't beat yourself up. Just get back to your good habits and follow the rules.

(Courtesy of UW Health Bariatric Surgery Program,
© 2008 University of Wisconsin Hospitals and Clinics Authority)

Foods: Glycemic Index

The glycemic index (GI) of a food is a measure of its effect on our blood sugar levels, which rise after we eat foods containing carbohydrates. It's a measurement of the speed at which a specific type of carbohydrate raises blood sugar. Only foods that contain carbohydrates have a GI. Foods containing little or no carbohydrate (such as meat, fish, eggs, avocado, and most vegetables) have no GI value.

The number is based on a comparison with glucose, which has a GI of 100. The lower the GI of a food, the better for sustaining weight loss (because it's better at controlling our appetite and delaying hunger) and reducing our risk of heart disease and diabetes.

The GI for many foods will vary: for fruits, vegetables, and dairy products, according to the type or variety and source; for processed foods, particularly according to the amounts of sugar and refined flour they contain. (Of course, the GI has no relation to calories!)

To check the GI of foods, visit *www.glycemicindex.com.*

Foods in Alphabetical Order, by Groups

BREADS

Bagel 72
Bread, sourdough 52
Bread, whole grain, pumpernickel 46
Bread, whole grain, rye 62
Bread, white wheat flour 70
Bread, whole wheat 69
Kaiser roll 73

CEREALS

All-Bran®, Kellogg's 42
Cheerios®, General Mills 74
Corn Flakes®, Kellogg's 83
Cream of Wheat®, B&G 66
Grape-Nuts®, Post 67
Grape-Nuts Flakes®, Post 80
Oatmeal 61
Puffed Rice®, Quaker 95

Puffed Wheat®, Quaker 74
Rice Krispies®, Kellogg's 82
Shredded Wheat®, Post 69
Special K®, Kellogg's 69
Total®, General Mills 76

GRAINS

Barley 25
Bulgur 48
Rice, brown 55
Rice, converted 47
Rice, instant 87
Rice, white 56

PASTA

Macaroni, regular 46
Spaghetti, regular 41
Spaghetti, whole wheat 37

BEANS AND NUTS

Almonds 0
Beans, baked 48
Beans, cooked 29
Beans, kidney, boiled 42
Beans, navy, boiled 30
Beans, pinto, boiled 39
Beans, red, boiled 28
Cashews 22
Chickpeas/Garbanzo beans 33
Lentils 29
Peanuts 14
Pecans 0
Soybeans 18
Walnuts 15

VEGETABLES

Beets 66
Broccoli 10
Cabbage 10

Carrots 49
Corn, sweet 55
Lettuce 10
Mushrooms 10
Onions 10
Parsnips 97
Peas, green 48
Peppers, red 10
Potato, new 62
Potato, sweet 52
Potato, white, baked 85
Pumpkin 75

FRUIT

Apple 36
Banana 52
Cantaloupe 65
Grapefruit 25
Grapes 46
Mango 55
Orange 43
Peach 28
Peaches, canned 47
Pear 36
Pineapple 66
Plum 39
Raisins 64
Strawberries 40
Watermelon 72

DAIRY PRODUCTS

Ice cream, low-fat (1.2 % fat) 47
Ice cream, regular 61
Milk, chocolate 34
Milk, skim 32
Milk, whole 27
Yogurt, low-fat 33
Yogurt, low-fat, fruit 33
Yogurt, regular 36

BEVERAGES

Juice, apple, unsweetened 40
Juice, grapefruit, unsweetened 48
Juice, orange 52
Juice, pineapple, unsweetened 46
Juice, tomato, canned,
   no added sugar 38

SNACKS

Chips, corn 72
Chips, potato chips 54

Chocolate bar 68
Crackers, soda 74
Jelly beans 80
Popcorn 55
Rice cakes 82
Rye crisp bread 63

SWEETENERS

Honey 58
Sugar, table (sucrose) 65

Foods in Order of GI

0 Almonds
0 Pecans
10 Broccoli
10 Cabbage
10 Lettuce
10 Mushrooms
10 Onions
10 Peppers, red
14 Peanuts
15 Walnuts
18 Soybeans
22 Cashews
25 Barley
25 Grapefruit
27 Milk, whole
28 Beans, red, boiled
28 Peach
29 Beans, cooked
29 Lentils
30 Beans, navy, boiled
32 Milk, skim
33 Chickpeas/Garbanzo beans
33 Yogurt, low-fat
33 Yogurt, low-fat fruit

34 Milk, chocolate
36 Apple
36 Pear
36 Yogurt, regular
37 Spaghetti, whole wheat
38 Juice, tomato, canned,
    no added sugar
39 Beans, pinto, boiled
39 Plum
40 Juice, apple, unsweetened
40 Strawberries
41 Spaghetti, regular
42 All-Bran®, Kellogg's
42 Beans, kidney, boiled
43 Bread, whole grain,
    pumpernickel
43 Orange
46 Grapes
46 Juice, pineapple, unsweetened
46 Macaroni, regular
47 Ice cream, low-fat (1.2 % fat)
47 Peaches, canned
47 Rice, converted
48 Beans, baked

48 Bulgur	66 Pineapple
48 Juice, grapefruit, unsweetened	67 Grape-Nuts®, Post
48 Peas, green	68 Chocolate bar
49 Carrots	69 Bread, whole wheat
52 Banana	69 Shredded Wheat®, Post
52 Bread, sourdough	69 Special K®, Kellogg's
52 Juice, orange	70 Bread, white wheat flour
52 Sweet potato	72 Bagel
54 Chips, potato	72 Chips, corn
55 Mango	72 Watermelon
55 Popcorn	73 Kaiser roll
55 Rice, brown	74 Cheerios®, General Mills
55 Sweet corn	74 Crackers, soda
56 Rice, white	74 Puffed Wheat®, Quaker
58 Honey	75 Pumpkin
61 Ice cream, regular	76 Total®, General Mills
61 Oatmeal	80 Grape-Nuts Flakes®, Post
62 Bread, whole grain, rye	80 Jelly beans
62 Potato, new	82 Rice cakes
63 Rye crisp bread	82 Rice Krispies®, Kellogg's
64 Beets	83 Corn Flakes®, Kellogg's
64 Raisins	85 Potato, white, baked
65 Cantaloupe	87 Rice, instant
65 Sugar, table (sucrose)	95 Puffed Rice®, Quaker
66 Cream of Wheat®, B&G	97 Parsnips

Glycemic Load

The carbohydrates we eat are rarely pure; they're combined in our foods with protein, fat, and indigestible fiber. To measure the impact of carbohydrates on our blood sugar levels more accurately, we can calculate the glycemic load (GL) of foods. This is especially important when the carbohydrate in a food has a high GI. Many foods have a high GI but a low GL, including carrots, parsnips, watermelon, broad beans, and pumpkin. You can compare GIs and GLs on the Revised International Table of Glycemic Index (GI) and Glycemic Load (GL), 2002: *www.mendosa.com/gilists.htm.*

Resources

Books

Weight Loss Surgery: Finding the Thin Person Hiding Inside You
Barbara Thompson (Word Association Publishers, 3rd edition, 2003)

Smart Exercise: Burning Fat, Getting Fit
Covert Bailey (Houghton Mifflin, 1994)

Power of 10: The Once-a-Week Slow Motion Fitness Revolution
Adam Zickerman and Bill Schley (Quill/HarperCollins
Publishers, 2004)

Breaking Free from Emotional Eating
Geneen Roth (Plume, 2003)

*When Food Is Love: Exploring the Relationship
Between Eating and Intimacy*
Geneen Roth (Plume, 1992)

Feeding the Hungry Heart: The Experience of Compulsive Eating
Geneen Roth (Plume Books, 1993)

Why Weight? A Guide to Ending Compulsive Eating
Geneen Roth (Plume Books, 1989)

Mindless Eating: Why We Eat More Than We Think
Brian Wansink, Ph.D. (Bantam Publishing, 2006)

*The Ten Habits of Naturally Slim People
and How to Make Them Part of Your Life*
Jill H. Podjasek with Jennifer Carney (Contemporary Books, 1998)

The Solution: 6 Winning Ways to Permanent Weight Loss
Laurel Mellin (HarperCollins Books, 1997)

The Success Habits of Weight-Loss Surgery Patients
Colleen M. Cook (Bariatric Support Centers International, 2003)

*The Success Habits of Weight-Loss Surgery Patients:
Final Success Workbook*
Colleen M. Cook (Bariatric Support Centers International, 2004)

Before and After: Living and Eating Well After Weight-Loss Surgery
Susan Maria Leach (William Morrow Cookbooks,
revised edition, 2004)

*Eating Well After Weight Loss Surgery:
Over 140 Delicious Low-Fat High-Protein Recipes
to Enjoy in the Weeks, Months and Years After Surgery*
Patt Levine and Michele Bontempo-Saray
(Marlowe & Company, 2004)

*Recipes for Life After Weight-Loss Surgery:
Delicious Dishes for Nourishing the New You*
Margaret Furtado and Lynette Schultz (Fair Winds Press, 2007)

Cookin' for Weight Loss Surgery Patients
Dick Stucki (Bonneville Publishing Co., 2005)

Weight-Loss Surgery Patient to Patient Cookbook
Bariatric Support Centers International
www.bariatricsupportcenter.com

*Your Erroneous Zones: Step-by-Step Advice for Escaping
the Trap of Negative Thinking and Taking Control of Your Life*
Wayne W. Dyer (Time Warner Paperbacks, 2005)

Taming Your Gremlin
Rick Carson (Collins, revised edition, 2003)

Culinary Classics: Essentials of Cooking
for the Gastric Bypass Patient
David Fouts (U.S. Bariatric, 2003)

Weight Loss Surgery for Dummies
Marina S. Kurian, Barbara Thompson, and Brian K. Davidson
(Wiley Publishing, 2005)

The Emotional First Aid Kit:
A Practical Guide to Life After Bariatric Surgery
Cynthia L. Alexander (Matrix Medical Communications, 2006)

Obesity Surgery: Stories of Altered Lives
Marta Meana and Lindsey Ricciardi (University of
Nevada Press, 2008)

Magazine

WLS Lifestyles, quarterly (DDB Media LLC), *www.wlslifestyles.com*

Web Sites

American Society for Metabolic and Bariatric Surgery
www.asmbs.org

Bariatric Surgery, UW Health, University of Wisconsin
Hospital, Madison
www.uwhealth.org/weightlosssurgery/madisonwisconsin/10410

ObesityHelp
www.obesityhelp.com

ObesityHelp Nutrition Forum
www.obesityhelp.com/forums/nutrition

Dietary Guidelines for Post-Bariatric Surgery (RD411.com)
www.rd411.com/article.php?ID=17

Living Well After WLS
www.livingafterwls.com/Recipes.html

ObesityHelp Forums
www.obesityhelp.com/forums

Support and Advice for Weight-Loss Surgery
groups.msn.com/SupportAdviceforWeightLossSurgeryMessageBoard

Obesity Discussion Forums
www.obesitydiscussion.com/forums

ThinnerTimes — Gastric Bypass and Lap-Band® Forum
www.thinnertimesforum.com

Home of the Glycemic Index
www.glycemicindex.com

Revised International Table of Glycemic Index and Glycemic Load, 2002 *www.mendosa.com/gilists.htm*

The Center for Mindful Eating
www.tcme.org

Co-active Coaching (life coaching)
www.co-activenetwork.com

Fearless Living (life coaching)
www.fearlessliving.org

UW Health Bariatric Surgery Program discussion board
www.meriter.com/living/discussion

Bariatric Eating — products, resources, and recipes
www.bariatriceating.com

Bariatric Support Centers International —
resources and support information
www.bariatricsupportcenter.com

Vitalady — products and resources for bariatric surgery
www.vitalady.com

CPSIA information can be obtained at www.ICGtesting.com
Printed in the USA
BVOW071732161212

308348BV00001B/177/P